SECOND EDITION
FITNESSGRAM®

Test Administration Manual

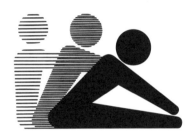

Developed by:
The Cooper Institute for Aerobics Research
Dallas, Texas

Primary Authors:
Marilu D. Meredith, EdD, Project Director
Gregory J. Welk, PhD, Scientific Director

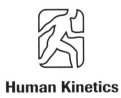

Human Kinetics

ISBN: 0-7360-0112-3

This book is a revised edition of *The Prudential FITNESSGRAM Test Administration Manual,* published in 1994 by The Cooper Institute for Aerobics Research.

Acquisitions Editor: Scott Wikgren; **Managing Editor:** Jennifer Clark; **Copyeditor:** Sarah Wiseman; **Proofreader:** Debra Aglaia; **Graphic Designer:** Nancy Rasmus; **Graphic Artist:** Denise Lowry; **Cover Designer:** Jack W. Davis; **Illustrators:** Tim Offenstein and Denise Lowry; **Printer:** Versa

Printed in the United States of America   10   9   8   7   6   5   4   3   2   1

Human Kinetics
Web site: http://www.humankinetics.com/

United States: Human Kinetics, P.O. Box 5076, Champaign, IL 61825-5076
1-800-747-4457
e-mail: humank@hkusa.com

Canada: Human Kinetics, 475 Devonshire Road Unit 100, Windsor, ON N8Y 2L5
1-800-465-7301 (in Canada only)
e-mail: humank@hkcanada.com

Europe: Human Kinetics, P.O. Box IW14, Leeds LS16 6TR, United Kingdom
(44) 1132 781708
e-mail: humank@hkeurope.com.com

Australia: Human Kinetics, 57A Price Avenue, Lower Mitcham, South Australia 5062
(088) 277 1555
e-mail: humank@hkaustralia.com

New Zealand: Human Kinetics, P.O. Box 105-231, Auckland 1
(09) 523 3462
e-mail: humank@hknewz.com

Contents

Acknowledgments

The current version of *FITNESSGRAM* is the fourth revision of our youth fitness reporting system. Since the last version, many significant developments have occurred in the physical education field. In 1996, the Surgeon General's Report on Physical Activity and Health was released. This provided strong documentation on the importance of physical activity for all segments of the population, especially children. In 1997, the Centers for Disease Control and Prevention released their Guidelines for School and Community Programs to Promote Lifelong Physical Activity Among Young People. In 1998, the Council for Physical Education for Children (COPEC) released a statement on appropriate physical activity for children. Collectively, these developments provide physical educators and youth fitness promoters with considerable support and guidelines to promote physical activity and fitness in children. The new version of *FITNESSGRAM* was designed to keep pace with these developments and to keep you on the cutting edge of youth fitness promotion. The final product is the result of cooperative efforts of many individuals.

Sincere appreciation is extended to the following persons who serve on the *FITNESSGRAM* Advisory Committee. Many dedicated hours were spent in the development and refinement of the total program.

Dr. Steven N. Blair, The Cooper Institute for Aerobics Research
Dr. Charles B. Corbin, Arizona State University
Dr. Kirk J. Cureton, The University of Georgia
Dr. Harold B. Falls, Jr., Southwest Missouri State University
Dr. Timothy G. Lohman, The University of Arizona
Dr. James R. Morrow, Jr., The University of North Texas
Dr. Robert P. Pangrazi, Arizona State University
Dr. Russell R. Pate, The University of South Carolina
Dr. Sharon A. Plowman, Northern Illinois University
Dr. James F. Sallis, San Diego State University
Dr. Charles L. Sterling, The Cooper Institute for Aerobics Research

Staff at The Cooper Institute for Aerobics Research including Mrs. Rhonda Carter, Mrs. Kelly Wilks, and Mr. Jay Weesner have also contributed significantly to refining and finalizing details of this version of *FITNESSGRAM*. Special recognition is in order for Dr. Charles Sterling, founder of the *FITNESSGRAM*, who continues to provide creative leadership and guidance for the program.

Dr. Marilu D. Meredith—Project Director
Dr. Gregory J. Welk—Scientific Director

Part

I

FITNESSGRAM

Chapter **1** About *FITNESSGRAM*

FITNESSGRAM is a comprehensive health-related fitness and activity assessment and computerized reporting system. All elements within *FITNESSGRAM* are designed to assist teachers in accomplishing the primary objective of youth fitness programs, which is to help students establish physical activity as a part of their daily lives.

The goals of *FITNESSGRAM* are to promote enjoyable regular physical activity and to provide comprehensive physical fitness and activity assessments and reporting programs for children and youth. *FITNESSGRAM* seeks to develop affective, cognitive, and behavioral components related to participation in regular physical activity in all children and youth, regardless of gender, age, disability, or any other factor. We believe that regular physical activity contributes to good health, function, and well-being and is important throughout a person's lifetime. Therefore, school programs should have the long-term view of promoting appropriate physical activity rather than focusing only on testing and performance aspects of physical fitness in children and youth. *FITNESSGRAM* emphasizes participation in a wide variety of physical activities to develop and maintain an acceptable level of physical fitness. We endorse the concept that physical activity should be fun and enjoyable.

Health-related physical fitness involves several components: aerobic capacity; body composition; and muscular strength, endurance, and flexibility. An appropriate physical activity program will address all of these elements. Whereas other physical fitness programs in the past have emphasized the attainment of high levels of performance on components of fitness, we believe strongly that extremely high levels of physical fitness, while admirable, are not necessary to accomplish objectives associated with good health and improved function. We believe it is important for all children to have adequate levels of activity and fitness. In a free society, individuals choose what they want to emphasize and where they want to strive for excellence. Some students will decide to make such an effort in music, art, or drama; others, for example, athletes, will give high priority to physical activity and fitness. We recognize this as proper, and want *FITNESSGRAM* to help all children and youth achieve a level of activity and fitness associated with excellent health, growth, and function.

Chapter 2 ∣ Fitness Education Guidelines

This section summarizes a process for conducting a physical fitness education program. *FITNESSGRAM* is an appropriate assessment tool to use in this process. Physical education teachers are encouraged to make use of other guidelines as well (Council for Physical Education for Children 1998, National Association for Sport and Physical Education 1995, Centers for Disease Control and Prevention 1997) and resources (*Physical Best*, Human Kinetics, physical education books by Pate) when planning their program (see reference list). A detailed discussion (and recommendation) on the role of physical education is provided in chapter 10.

Short-Term Objective

The short-term objective of a physical fitness educational program is to provide students with opportunities to learn fitness concepts while participating in enjoyable activities that enhance fitness levels.

Long-Term Objective

The long-term objective of a physical fitness educational program is to teach students the skills they need to be active for life. Students should learn to self-assess their fitness levels, interpret assessment results, plan personal programs, and motivate themselves to remain active on their own. With regular physical activity all students should be able to achieve a score that will place them within or above the Healthy Fitness Zone on all *FITNESSGRAM* test items.

The Fitness Process Step by Step

Step One: Instruction About Fitness Foundation Concepts

Students should be instructed in basic concepts of fitness development and maintenance. Concepts should include the following areas:

- Importance of regular exercise for health and the prevention of degenerative diseases
- Description of each area of fitness and its importance to health
- Methods to use in developing each area of fitness

Step Two: Student Participation in Conditioning Activities

Students should be preconditioned for testing to maximize safety. The Get Fit program provided in appendix C may be used for this purpose. Do some of these activities in class; assign others for completion during student's leisure.

Step Three: Instruction on Test Items

Include the following topics when teaching each test item:

- What it measures
- How to administer it
- Practice sessions

Step Four: Assessment of Fitness Levels

If possible, allow students to test one another or have a team of parents assist in conducting the assessments. Also, teach students to conduct self-assessment.

Step Five: Planning the Fitness Program and Setting Goals

After completing the fitness tests, use the results to help each student set goals and plan his or her personal fitness program. Be sure to include the following activities:

- Inform students and parents of results with *FITNESSGRAM* report.
- Teach students how to interpret their results.
- Assist students in setting process goals for an exercise program that will improve or maintain their fitness levels (see appendix C for goal-setting form).
- Evaluate group performance.

Step Six: Promotion and Tracking of Physical Activity

The teacher or fitness leader should make every effort to motivate students to establish regular physical activity habits and to recognize them for success in their efforts. The *ACTIVITYGRAM* program provides an ideal way to help students track their physical activity.

Allow time during physical education for students to work toward their goals. You should also expect them to spend some of their leisure time participating in fun activities that will help them achieve their goals. The critical consideration is that students should have FUN while participating in physical activity.

Step Seven: Reassessment

Periodic reassessment of students' fitness levels apprises students of how they are changing and reinforces for them the practice of "sticking with it." When you report their results, show the progress of individuals using *FITNESSGRAM* and of the group using a *FITNESSGRAM* statistical report. Recognition for achieving goals is a vital part of establishing behavior patterns.

Step Eight: Revision

Reassessment yields new information so that we can revise or refine our goals, when desirable, in keeping with the emerging picture. In planning adjustments of your activity program, keep in mind that your students will benefit not only from your plans tailored for them but also from your teaching them how to revise their own fitness goals and from ongoing instruction in fitness concepts.

Chapter ∎3∎ Physical Fitness Testing

FITNESSGRAM is designed to evaluate and educate youth about the status of their physical fitness. This information can be used in different ways depending on the teacher's, school's, or agency's philosophy of fitness evaluation. Various testing procedures are possible depending on the primary objective of the program.

Provide Information on Individual Fitness Level

One of the primary objectives of fitness testing is to provide the student, teacher, and parents with personal information regarding the student's current level of fitness. The information regarding fitness status can then be used as the basis for designing personal, individualized programs of fitness development. When the purpose of testing is to provide students with personal information, several approaches may be used in conducting the assessments.

• **Traditional:** The traditional approach is to have the teacher or a trained adult conduct the assessments on each student. Attention is focused on correct protocol, and teacher interaction is included to motivate students to achieve their best performance.

• **Self-testing:** A more contemporary focus is on self-testing. In this approach students learn the process and concepts of fitness testing so that they will be able to evaluate their fitness status throughout life. This approach is student-centered. Students are asked to select a testing partner; the two work together to evaluate each other's fitness. Students are encouraged to perform at their own personal best level. Testing stations are established, and students rotate from one station to another to complete the evaluation. Teachers should provide encouragement and praise for correct testing procedure as well as performance. The results are used in class to allow the student to monitor progress throughout the term of the class.

• **Criterion-based self-testing:** In some situations teachers may elect to have students stop the test when they have achieved a score equal to the upper limit of the Healthy Fitness Zone. Stopping the test performance in this manner can reduce required testing time. It may also reduce the possibility of embarrassment and avoid creating a threatening environment caused by assessments for students who are less capable. If this approach is used, parents should be informed about the process so that they understand that the performance reported on *FITNESSGRAM* does not necessarily represent a maximal effort. Also, if performance during class time does not allow a maximal effort, it is good to provide those more highly motivated students the opportunity to do a maximal test at some other time. An after-school fitness challenge may prove to be very popular with students who are high-level performers.

With the *FITNESSGRAM* software several options are also possible for how the fitness reports are generated.

• **Teacher-entered data:** Teachers can enter scores into the teacher version of the software. The software allows quick spreadsheet-like data entry to speed up data-entry tasks.

• **Student-entered data:** Students can enter their own scores into the student version of the software. The interactive software allows students to learn more about fitness and the importance of physical activity. By entering their own scores, students will also learn that fitness is personal. Because of the educational value for students, we advocate that students enter their own data.

Provide Information for Program Evaluation

A second objective of fitness assessment may be to determine whether the program is achieving its stated goals. If the curriculum or program is adequate, the students should be achieving institutional goals. A common approach is to establish a percentage of the student body that should achieve the Healthy Fitness Zone or above. If the resulting percentage is below the stated goal, emphasis in the curriculum may need to be adjusted in order to increase the number of students achieving the goal.

Testing for program evaluation should be done in a formal manner. A suggested approach is to train a group of volunteers to assist the teacher in administering test items. Scores are entered into the computer, and then a statistical report can be run to determine the percentage of students achieving the Healthy Fitness Zone.

Chapter 4 FITNESSGRAM Test Administration

The *FITNESSGRAM* assessment measures three components of physical fitness which have been identified as being important because of their relationship to overall health and optimal function. The three components are aerobic capacity; body composition; and muscular strength, endurance, and flexibility. Several test options are provided for most areas, with one test item being recommended. This chapter describes procedures for administering and scoring test items. Appendix C contains samples of class scoresheets or individual scoresheets for self-assessment. The *FITNESSGRAM* software will also print a class scoresheet. Table 4.1 provides a summary list of the test items.

A new feature of *FITNESSGRAM*, Revision 6.0, is the inclusion of physical activity assessments. These assessments were added because we need to reinforce for children the importance of developing lifetime habits of regular physical activity. While fitness is important, it cannot be maintained unless children are physically active.

One opportunity to assess physical activity patterns within the *FITNESSGRAM* program is the *FITNESSGRAM* Physical Activity Questionnaire. In order to use the *FITNESSGRAM* Physical Activity Questionnaire, you must have the student application installed and allow the student to enter their own information.

Considerations for Testing Primary Grades

The major emphasis when testing children in grades K-3 should be on enjoyment and instructions on proper technique. It is important at this level not to focus on level of performance. Performance standards are not available for the aerobic capacity test items for students younger than 10 years of age. While standards are provided for other test items for primary grade children, you are strongly encouraged not to emphasize performance level and test results.

Table 4.1 *FITNESSGRAM* Test Items

Aerobic Capacity

Teachers will select one of the following options:
 *The PACER
 One-mile run
 The walk test (secondary students)

Body Composition

Teachers may select one of the following options:
 *Skinfold measurements
 Body mass index

Muscle Strength, Endurance, and Flexibility

Teachers will select as indicated

Abdominal Strength and Endurance

Must select.
 *Curl-up

Trunk Extensor Strength and Flexibility

Must select.
 *Trunk lift

Upper Body Strength

Must select one.
 *Push-up
 Modified pull-up
 Pull-up
 Flexed arm hang

Flexibility

May select one.
 Back-saver sit and reach
 Shoulder stretch

---

*Recommended test.

Safety Considerations

The test items used in *FITNESSGRAM* have been administered to millions of students and have proven to be very safe. The prudent teacher, however, will recognize that with any strenuous physical activity there is always the possibility that incidents may occur.

Prior to administering any test items, it is vital that you be aware of the potential health problems of all students in your classes. It is possible that a student could have a congenital heart condition that may require special consideration during the administration of an aerobic capacity measure or other test items. Maximizing the safety of all students should be a primary objective.

Your school district or agency should have established policies related to medical information, medical records, and medical clearance for activity. It is important that you be aware of these policies and that you follow them strictly.

AEROBIC CAPACITY

Aerobic capacity is perhaps the most important area of any fitness program. Research clearly indicates that acceptable levels of aerobic capacity are associated with a reduced risk of high blood pressure, coronary heart disease, obesity, diabetes, some forms of cancer and other health problems in adults (Blair et al. 1989, Blair et al. 1992).

Aerobic capacity relative to body weight is considered to be the best indicator of a person's overall cardiorespiratory capacity. Many terms have been used to describe this dimension of physical fitness, including cardiovascular fitness, cardiorespiratory fitness, cardiorespiratory endurance, aerobic fitness, aerobic work capacity, and physical working capacity. Although defined somewhat differently, these terms can generally be considered to be synonymous with aerobic capacity. A laboratory measure of maximal oxygen uptake ($\dot{V}O_2$max) is generally considered to be the best measure of aerobic capacity. The field tests used for aerobic capacity have demonstrated strong reliability and validity against measured $\dot{V}O_2$max (see the *FITNESSGRAM* Technical Reference Manual at the American Fitness Alliance website **http://www.americanfitness.net**).

In addition to the achieved test score, the estimated $\dot{V}O_2$max adjusted according to kilogram of body weight per minute is also reported on the *FITNESSGRAM* program output. It is possible to compare results between different measures such as the PACER, the one-mile run, and the walk test. These are the three aerobic capacity test options. The PACER is the default item for all students and is strongly recommended for participants in grades K-3. The emphasis for testing in grades K-3 should be on fun, allowing the students to participate in a pleasant experience.

The PACER

Recommended

The PACER (Progressive Aerobic Cardiovascular Endurance Run) is a multistage fitness test adapted from the 20-meter shuttle run test published by Leger and Lambert (1982) and revised in 1988 (Leger et al.). The test is progressive; it is easy at the beginning and gets harder. Set to music, this test is a valid, fun alternative to the customary distance run test for measuring aerobic capacity. The PACER is recommended for all ages. Information on obtaining the music CD or tape can be found in appendix A.

Teachers of grades K-3 are strongly encouraged to use the PACER. When administering the test to these younger children, the emphasis should be to allow the children to have a good time while learning how to take this test and how to pace. Allow children to continue to run as long as they wish and as long as they are still enjoying the activity. Typically the test in grades K-3 will only last a few minutes. It is not desirable or necessary to make them run to exhaustion.

Test Objective: To run as long as possible back and forth across a 20-meter space at a specified pace which gets faster each minute.

Equipment/Facilities: A flat, non-slippery surface at least 20 m long, CD or cassette player with adequate volume, CD or audio cassette, measuring tape, marker cones, pencil, and copies of scoresheet

A or B (see appendix C) are required. Students should wear shoes with nonslip soles. Plan for each student to have a 40-60 in. wide space for running.

Test Instructions:

• Mark the 20 m (21 yd, 32 in.) course with marker cones to divide lanes and a tape or chalk line at each end. If using the audiotape, calibrate it by timing the 1 min test interval at the beginning of the tape. If the tape has stretched and the timing is off by more than half a second, obtain another copy of the tape. Make copies of scoresheet A for each group of students to be tested.

• Before test day, allow students to listen to several minutes of the tape so that they know what to expect. Students should then be allowed at least two practice sessions.

• Allow students to select a partner. Have students who are being tested line up behind the start line.

• The PACER CD has a music version and one with only the beeps. The PACER tape has two music versions and one beep-only version. Each version of the test will give a 5-second countdown and tell the students when to start.

• Students should run across the 20 m distance and touch the line with their foot by the time the beep sounds. At the sound of the beep, they turn around and run back to the other end. If some students get to the line before the beep, they must wait for the beep before running the other direction. Students continue in this manner until they fail to reach the line before the beep for the second time.

• A single beep will sound at the end of the time for each lap. A triple beep sounds at the end of each minute. The triple beep serves the same function as the single beep and also alerts the runners that the pace will get faster.

When to Stop: The first time a student does not reach the line by the beep, she reverses direction immediately. Allow a student to attempt to catch up with the pace. The test is completed for a student when she fails to reach the line by the beep for the *second* time. Students just completing the test should continue to walk and stretch in the cool-down area. Figure 4.1 provides diagrams of testing procedures.

Scoring: In the PACER test, a lap is one 20 m distance (from one end to the other). Have one student recording the lap number (crossing off each lap number) on a PACER score sheet (samples provided in appendix C). The recorded score is the total number of laps completed by the student. For ease in administration, count the first lap that the student does not reach the line by the beep. It is important to be consistent with all of the students and classes.

An alternative scoring method is available. This method does not eliminate students when they miss their second beep (Schiemer 1996). Using the PACER Scoresheet B, the teacher establishes two different symbols to be used in recording, such as a star for making the line by the beep and a triangle for not making the line. The recording partner then draws a star in the circle when the runner successfully makes the line by the beep and a triangle when the runner fails to make the line by the beep, simply making a record of what occurs. The runners can continue to participate until the leader stops the music or until they voluntarily stop running. To determine the score, find the second triangle (or whatever symbol was used). The number associated with the preceding star is the score. An example is provided in figure 4.2.

Students ages five to nine years in grades K-3 should not receive a score; they simply participate in the activity. Enter a score of 0 laps to indicate that they successfully participated in the PACER run. Nine-year-olds in grade four may receive a score. All ten-year-old students should receive a score regardless of grade level.

Performance standards for students in grades K-3 have purposefully not been established. There are concerns regarding the reliability and validity of the test results for very young children. Even with practice, it is difficult to ensure that young children will pace themselves appropriately and give a maximal effort. The object of the test for these younger students is simply to participate and learn about the test protocol.

Suggestions for Test Administration:

• The test CD or tape contains 21 levels (1 level per minute for 21 min). The CD or tape allows 9 seconds for running the distance during the first minute. The lap time decreases by approximately one-half second at each successive level. Calibrating the tape may help.

• A single beep indicates the end of a lap (one 20 m distance). The students run from one end to the other between each beep. Caution students not to begin too fast. The beginning speed is very slow. Nine seconds is allowed for running each 20 m lap during the first minute.

• Triple beeps at the end of each minute indicate the end of a level and an increase in speed. Students should be alerted that the speed will increase. When students hear the triple beeps they should turn around at the line and immediately continue running. Some students will have a tendency to hesitate when they hear the triple beeps.

• A student who cannot reach the line when the beep sounds should be given one more beep to attempt to regain the pace before withdrawing from the activity. The second time a student cannot reach the line by the beep, his or her test is completed.

• Groups of students may be tested at one time. Adult volunteers may be asked to help record scores.

• Each runner must be allowed a path 40-60 wide. It may work best to mark the course.

• If possible, to save time use two tapes and two cassette players. Rewind the first tape while the second group is running the tests, and so forth.

AEROBIC CAPACITY

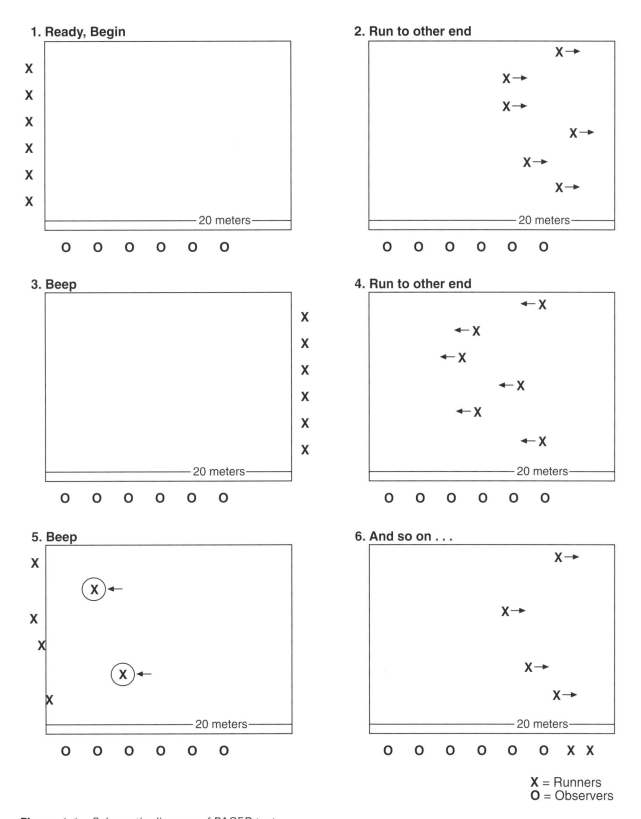

Figure 4.1   Schematic diagram of PACER test.

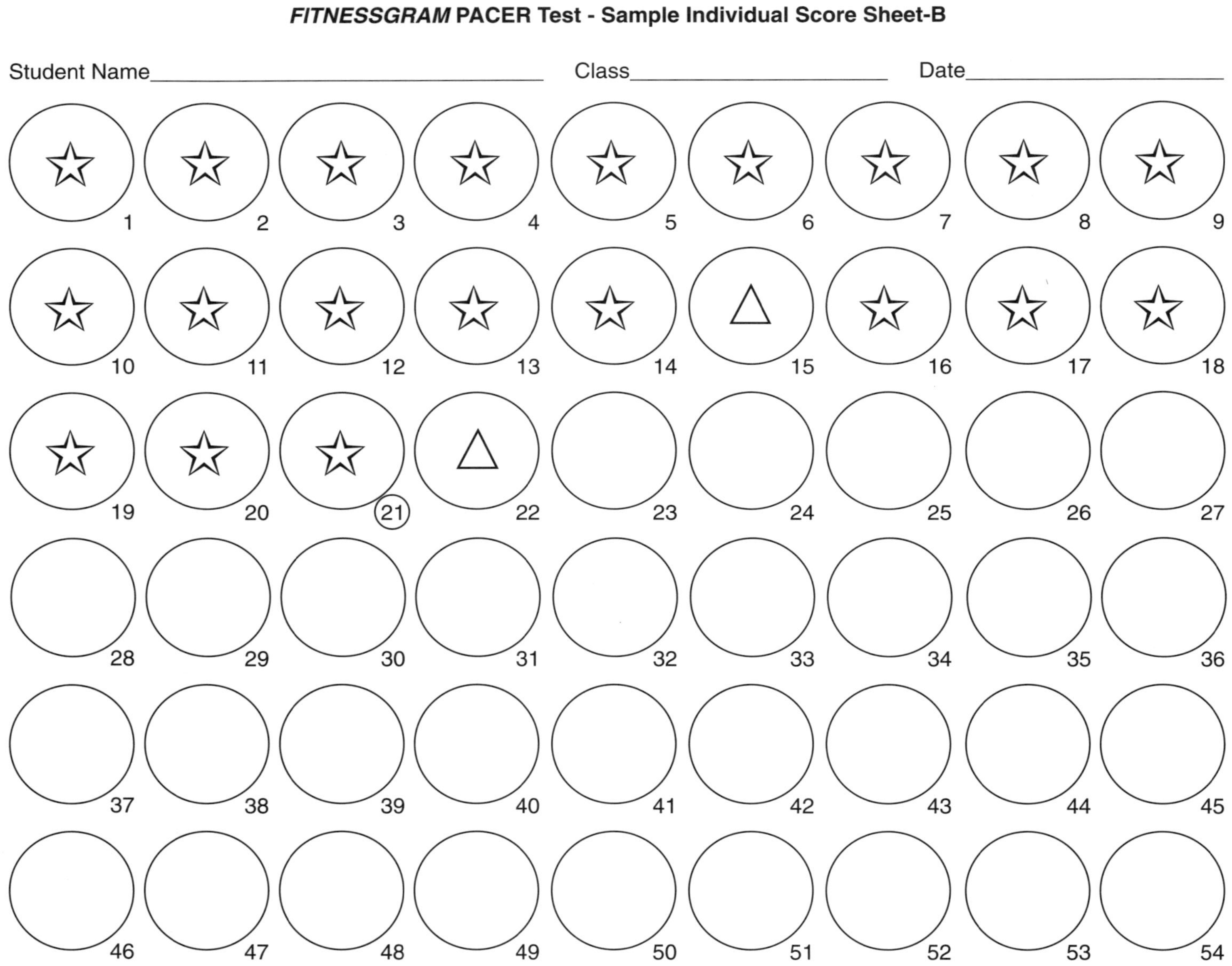

AEROBIC CAPACITY

FITNESSGRAM PACER Test - Sample Individual Score Sheet-B

Student Name _____ Class _____ Date _____

Figure 4.2 Stars for completed laps. Triangles for non-completed laps. Student's score would be 21.

AEROBIC CAPACITY

One-Mile Run

Alternative

Test Objective: The objective is to run a mile at the fastest pace possible. If a student cannot run the total distance, walking is permitted.

Equipment/Facilities: A flat running course, stopwatch, pencil, and scoresheets (included in appendix C) are required. The course may be a track or any other measured area. The course may be measured using a tape measure or cross country wheel. Caution: If the track is metric or shorter than 440 yd, adjust the running course (1,609.34 m = 1 mi; 400 m = 437.4 yd; 1,760 yd = 1 mi). On a metric track the run should be 4 laps plus 10 yd.

Test Instructions: Students begin on the signal "Ready, Start." As they cross the finish line, elapsed time should be called to the participants (or their partners). It is possible to test 15 to 20 students at one time by dividing the group and assigning partners. While one group runs, partners count laps and make note of finish time. Appendix C contains a sample scoresheet for partners to use.

Scoring: The one-mile run is scored in minutes and seconds. A score of 99 min and 99 s indicates that the student could not finish the distance. Students ages five to nine years in grades K-3 should not be timed; they should simply complete the distance and be given a score of 00 min and 00 s. Nine-year-olds in grade four may receive a score. All ten-year-olds should receive a score regardless of grade level.

Performance standards for students in grades K-3 have purposefully not been established. There are concerns regarding the reliability and validity of the test results for very young children. Even with practice, it is difficult to ensure that young children will pace themselves appropriately and give a maximal effort. The object of the test for these younger students is simply to complete the one mile distance at a comfortable pace and to practice pacing.

Suggestions for Test Administration:

• Preparation for the test should include instruction about pacing and practice in pacing. Without instruction, students will usually run too fast early in the test and then be forced to walk in the latter stages.

• Results are generally better if the student can maintain a constant pace during most of the test.

• Walking is definitely permitted. Although the objective is to cover the distance in the best possible time, students who must walk should not be made to feel inferior. Encourage students who walk to walk at a fast pace, rather than stroll. Attainment of the Healthy Fitness Zone is the important factor.

• Students should always warm up prior to taking the test. It is also important that students cool down by continuing to walk for several minutes after completing the distance.

• Administration of the test under conditions of unusually high temperature and/or humidity or when the wind is strong should be avoided as these elements may be unsafe or lead to an invalid estimate of aerobic capacity.

• Counting laps completed and accurately recording the run time can be a problem when a relatively small course is utilized with younger children. Many techniques are acceptable. Pair the students and have the resting partner count laps and record time for the runner. Older students or parents may be asked to assist in recording results for younger students. Appendix C contains a sample scoring and recording sheet.

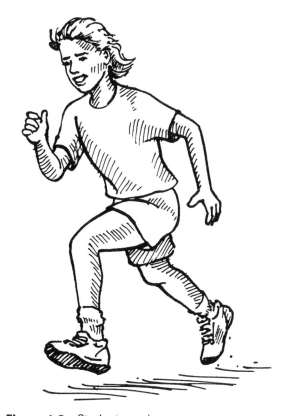

Figure 4.3   Student running.

AEROBIC CAPACITY

Walk Test

Alternative

Test Objective: The objective is to walk one mile as quickly as possible while maintaining a constant walking pace the entire distance. This test is included in *FITNESSGRAM* for use with participants ages 13 years and older. The walk test is an excellent self-assessment skill for everyone to use throughout their life.

Equipment/Facilities: A flat, measured running course, two or more stopwatches, pencils, and scoresheets (included in appendix C) are required. Heart rate monitors, if available, make heart rate monitoring much easier. The course may be measured using a tape measure or cross country wheel. Caution: If the track is metric or shorter than 440 yd, adjust the course (1,609.34 m = 1 mi; 400 m = 437.4 yd; 1,760 yd = 1 mi). On a metric track the run should be 4 laps plus 10 yd.

Test Instructions: Students begin on the signal "Ready, Start." Participants should attempt to walk the full mile as quickly as they can but at a pace that can be maintained the entire distance. As they cross the finish line, elapsed time should be called to the participants (or their partners). It is possible to test 15 to 30 students at one time by dividing the group and assigning partners. While one group walks, partners count laps and make note of finish time. Appendix C contains a sample scoresheet for partners to use.

At the conclusion of the one-mile walk, each student should take a 15-second heart rate. If using heart rate monitors, each participant starts his stopwatch at the beginning of the walk and stops it at the end. The last heart rate recorded during the walk is used as the walking heart rate unless it is less than 10 s, in which case one should use the heart rate taken as the watch is stopped at the end of the walk. If heart rate monitors are not used, many stopwatches or watches with second hands will be needed for timing heart rate. The participant should count his heart rate immediately after completing the mile. The observing partner can time the 15 s.

Scoring: The walk test is scored in minutes and seconds. A score of 99 min and 99 s indicates that the student could not finish the distance. A 15 s heart rate should be taken at the conclusion of the walk. Walk time and 15 s heart rate are entered in the *FITNESSGRAM* software. Estimated $\dot{V}O_2$max

is calculated using the Rockport Fitness Walking Test equation (Kline et al. 1987, McSwegin et al. 1998).

Suggestions for Test Administration:

• Preparation for the test should include instruction and practice in pacing and in techniques for heart rate monitoring.

• Results are generally better if the student can maintain a constant pace during most of the test.

• Students should always warm up prior to taking the test. It is also important that students cool down by continuing to walk for several minutes after completing the distance.

• Administration of the test under conditions of unusually high temperature and/or humidity or when the wind is strong should be avoided as these elements may cause an invalid estimate of aerobic capacity.

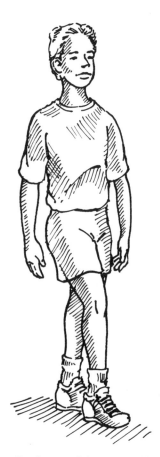

Figure 4.4   Student walking.

BODY COMPOSITION

The body composition test results provide an estimation of the percent of a student's weight that is fat in contrast to lean body mass (muscles, bones, organs). Maintaining appropriate body composition is vital in preventing the onset of obesity, which is associated with increased risk of coronary heart disease, stroke, and diabetes. Children and youth with levels greater than 25% fat for boys and 30% fat for girls are more likely to develop primary risk factors of heart disease, including high blood pressure and elevated cholesterol (Williams et al. 1992).

Research indicates that today's young people are fatter than in previous years (Pate et al. 1985, Gortmaker et al. 1987, Ross et al. 1987, Troiano 1998, Lohman 1992). The development of appropriate nutritional and behavioral patterns is important to reverse the trend of increasing fatness of our children and youth. A number of methods for estimating body composition in children and youth have been developed, including underwater weighing, total body water, anthropometry (skinfold measurement), bioelectrical impedence, and body mass index (height and weight). Each approach has some limitations leading to measurement errors of 2 to 3% in the estimate of percent fat. Estimates based on height and weight result in 5 to 6% error (Lohman 1987, Lohman 1992). Because of lower prediction error and the fact that skinfold measurements give a more direct estimate of body fatness than does body mass index, which also reflects muscle and bone mass, the recommended test option is the measurement of triceps and calf skinfolds. You can directly enter a calculated percent body fat with the *FITNESSGRAM* software so that you can use other assessment methods besides skinfold measurement or body mass index.

Skinfold Measurements

Recommended

Test Objective: To measure the triceps and calf skinfold thicknesses for calculating percent body fat.

Equipment/Facilities: A skinfold caliper is necessary to perform this measurement. The cost of calipers ranges from $5 to $200. Both the expensive and inexpensive calipers have been shown to be effective for use by teachers who have had sufficient training and practice. Appendix A lists sources for calipers.

Testing Procedures: The triceps and calf skinfolds have been chosen for *FITNESSGRAM* because they are easily measured and highly correlated with total body fatness. The caliper measures a double layer of subcutaneous fat and skin.

Measurement Location: The triceps skinfold is measured on the back of the arm over the triceps muscle of the right arm midway between the elbow and the acromion process of the scapula (figure 4.5). Using a piece of string to find the midpoint is a good suggestion. The skinfold site should be vertical. Pinching the fold slightly above the midpoint will ensure that the fold is measured right on the midpoint (figures 4.6 and 4.7).

The calf skinfold is measured on the inside of the right leg at the level of maximal calf girth. The right foot is placed flat on an elevated surface with the knee flexed at a 90° angle (figure 4.8). The vertical

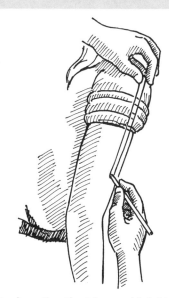

Figure 4.5   Locating the triceps skinfold site.

skinfold should be grasped just above the level of maximal girth (figure 4.9) and the measurement made below the grasp.

For college students, the formula to calculate percent body fat also includes the abdominal skinfold measurement in addition to the triceps and calf skinfolds. The abdominal skinfold is measured at a site 3 centimeters to the side of the midpoint of the

BODY COMPOSITION

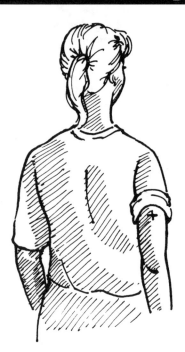

Figure 4.6 Site of the triceps skinfold.

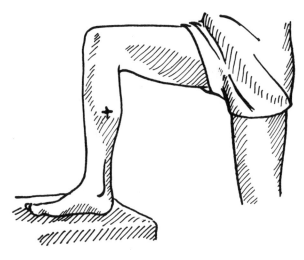

Figure 4.8 Placement of leg for locating the calf skinfold site.

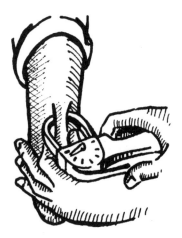

Figure 4.7 Triceps skinfold measurement.

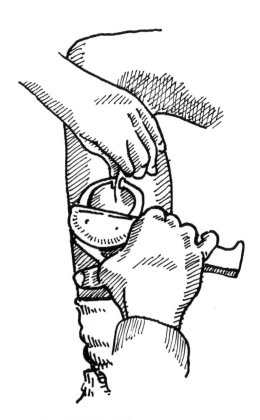

Figure 4.9 Calf skinfold measurement.

BODY COMPOSITION

umbilicus and 1 cm below it (figure 4.10). The skinfold is horizontal and should be measured on the right side of the body (figure 4.11) while the subject relaxes the abdominal wall as much as possible.

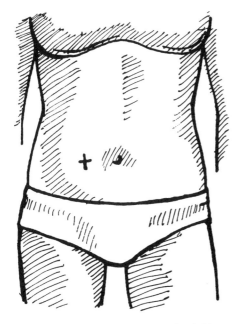

Figure 4.10 Site of abdominal skinfold.

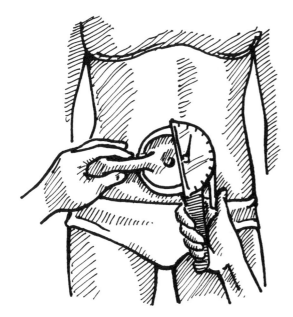

Figure 4.11 Abdominal skinfold measurement.

Measurement Technique:

- Measure skinfolds on the person's right side.
- Instruct the student to relax the arm or leg being measured.
- Firmly grasp the skinfold between the thumb and forefinger and lift it away from the other body tissue. The grasp should not be so firm as to be painful.
- Place the caliper 1/2 in. below the pinch site.
- Be sure the caliper is in the middle of the fold.
- The recommended procedure is to do one measurement at each site before doing the second measurement at each site and finally the third set of measurements.

Scoring: The skinfold measure is registered on the dial of the caliper. Each measurement should be taken three times, with the recorded score being the median (middle) value of the three scores. To illustrate: If the readings were 7.0, 9.0, and 8.0, the score would be recorded as 8.0 mm. Each reading should be recorded to the nearest 5 mm. For teachers not using the computer software, a percent fatness look-up chart is provided in appendix C.

Suggestions for Test Administration:

- Skinfolds should be measured in a setting that provides the child with privacy.
- Interpretation of the measurements may be given in a group setting as long as individual results are not identified.
- Whenever possible, it is recommended that the same tester administer the skinfold measurement to the same students at subsequent testing periods.
- Practice measuring the sites with another tester and compare results with the same students. As you become familiar with the methods you can generally find agreement within 10% between testers.

Learning to Do Skinfold Measurements: Using video training tapes or participating in a workshop are excellent ways to begin to learn how to do skinfold measurements. The videotape, *Measuring Body Fatness Using Skinfolds*, illustrates the procedures described in this manual. Appendix A contains information on obtaining this videotape.

BODY COMPOSITION

Body Mass Index

Alternative

The body mass index provides an indication of the appropriateness of a child's weight relative to height. Body mass index is determined by the following formula:

$$\text{Weight (kg)} / \text{Height}^2 \text{ (m)}.$$

While the data can be entered in pounds and inches, the results are only meaningful with the metric formula. For example, a student weighing 100 pounds (45.36 kg) who is 5 feet (1.52 m) tall would have a body mass index of 19.6. Another student of the same weight but 5 ft 2 in. tall would have a body mass index of 18.3.

Therefore, height and weight measures, recorded as a regular portion of the testing process for all students, are converted to metric units by the computer to calculate body mass index, pounds to kilograms and feet to meters. Body mass index is calculated only if skinfold measurements are not entered. Recommended body mass index scores are listed in chapter 5. A score which is classified as "Needs Improvement" generally indicates that a child weighs too much for his height. Body mass index is not the recommended procedure for determining body composition because it does not estimate the percent of fat. It merely provides information on the appropriateness of the weight relative to the height. For those children found to be too heavy for their height, a skinfold test would clarify whether the weight was due to excess fat.

MUSCLE STRENGTH, ENDURANCE, AND FLEXIBILITY

Tests of muscular strength, muscular endurance, and flexibility have been combined into one broad fitness category because the primary consideration is determining the health status of the musculoskeletal system. It is equally important to have strong muscles that can work forcefully and over a period of time and to be flexible enough to have a full range of motion at the joint. Musculoskeletal injuries are many times the result of muscle imbalance at a specific joint; the muscles on one side may be much stronger than the opposing muscles or may have inadequate flexibility to allow complete motion or sudden motion to occur.

It is important to remember that the specificity of training bears directly on the development of musculoskeletal strength, endurance, and flexibility. The movements included in these test items are only a sampling of the many ways that the body is required to move and adjust during physical activity.

The upper body and the abdominal/trunk region have been selected as areas for testing because of their perceived relationship to maintaining functional health and correct posture, thereby reducing possibilities of future low back pain and restrictions in independent living. Although most students will not have weaknesses sufficient to cause current problems, it is important to educate them regarding the importance of muscle strength, endurance, and flexibility in preventing problems as adults. It is especially important to make students aware of correct postural alignment and body mechanics in the event that they are developing scoliosis, which is a problem for teenage youth. The school nurse, a local physician, or a physical therapist is a good source of information about scoliosis.

The curl-up and the push-up have been adapted from assessments reported by Massicote (1990).

Abdominal Strength and Endurance

Strength and endurance of the abdominal muscles are important in promoting good posture and correct pelvic alignment. The latter is particularly important in the maintenance of low back health. In testing and training the muscles of this region it is difficult to isolate the abdominal muscles. The modified sit-up, which was used previously, involves the action of the hip flexor muscles in addition to the abdominal muscles. The curl-up has been selected because it does not involve the assistance of the hip flexor muscles and minimizes compression in the spine, when compared to a full sit-up with the feet held.

Curl-Up

Recommended

Test Objective: To complete as many curl-ups as possible up to a maximum of 75 at a specified pace.

Equipment/Facilities: Gym mats and a measuring strip for every two students are needed. The measuring strip may be made of cardboard, rubber, smooth wood, or any similar thin flat material and should be 30 to 35 inches long. Two widths of measuring strip may be needed. The narrower strip should be 3 in. wide and is used to test 5- to 9-year-olds; for older students the strip should be 4 1/2 in. wide. Other methods of measuring distance such as using tape strips and pencils are suggested in appendix A.

Test Instructions: Allow students to select a partner. Partner A will perform the curl-ups while partner B counts and watches for form errors.

Partner A lies in a supine position on the mat, knees bent at an angle of approximately 140°, feet flat on the floor, legs slightly apart, arms straight and parallel to the trunk with palms of hands resting on the mat. The fingers are stretched out and the head is in contact with the mat.

After partner A has assumed the correct position on the mat, partner B places a measuring strip on the mat under the legs so that fingertips are just resting on the nearest edge of the measuring strip (figure 4.12). Partner B then kneels down at partner A's head in a position to count curl-ups and watch for form breaks. Partner B may place hands under partner A's head or a piece of paper may be put on the mat instead to help partner B see that partner A's head touched down on each repetition

MUSCLE STRENGTH, ENDURANCE, AND FLEXIBILITY

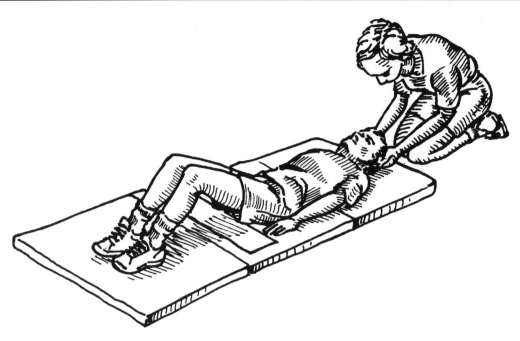

Figure 4.12 Starting position for the curl-up test.

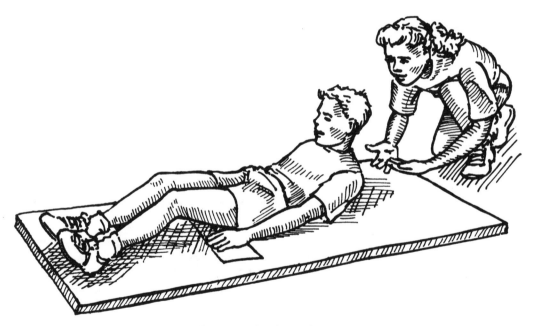

Figure 4.13 Position of student in the "up" position for the curl-up test.

(figure 4.13). Watch for the paper to crinkle each time partner A touches it with her head.

Keeping heels in contact with the mat partner A curls up slowly, sliding fingers across the measuring strip until fingertips reach the other side (figures 4.14a and b), then curls back down until his head touches the mat. Movement should be slow and gauged to the specified cadence of about 20 curl-ups per minute (one curl every 3 seconds).

The teacher should call a cadence or use a pre-recorded cadence. A recorded cadence may be found on the PACER music tape or CD. Partner A continues without pausing until he can no longer continue or has completed 75 curl-ups.

When to Stop: Students are stopped after completing 75 curl-ups or when the second form correction is made.

MUSCLE STRENGTH, ENDURANCE, AND FLEXIBILITY

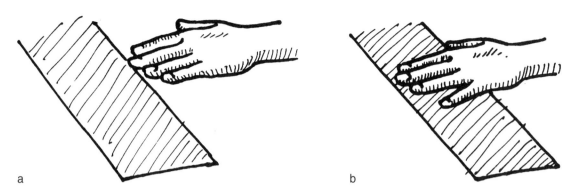

a   b

Figures 4.14a and 4.14b   Close-up of fingertips sliding from one side of the measuring strip to the other.

Scoring: The score is the number of curl-ups performed. Count should be made when the student's head returns to the mat. For ease in administration, it is permissible to count the first incorrect curl-up. It is important to be consistent with all of the students and classes.

Form Corrections:

- Heels must remain in contact with the mat.
- Head must return to the mat on each repetition.
- Pauses and rest periods are not allowed. The movement should be continuous and with the cadence.
- Fingertips should touch the far side of the measuring strip.

Suggestions for Test Administration:

- The student being tested should reposition if the body moves so that the head does not contact the mat at the appropriate spot or the measuring strip is out of position.
- Movement should start with a flattening of the lower back followed by a slow curling of the upper spine.
- The hands should slide across the measuring

strip until the fingertips reach the opposite side (3 or 4 1/2 in.) and then return to the supine position. The movement is completed when the back of the head touches the partner's hand.

- The cadence will encourage a steady, continuous movement done in the correct form.
- Students should not "reach" with their arms and hands but simply let the arms passively move along the floor in response to the action of the trunk and shoulders. Any jerking or reaching motion will cause the students to constantly move out of position.
- This curl-up protocol is quite different from the one-minute sit-up. Students will need to learn the correct form for this skill and be allowed time to practice.

Trunk Extensor Strength and Flexibility

A test of trunk extensor strength and flexibility is being included in *FITNESSGRAM* because of its relationship to low back health, especially proper vertebral alignment. Musculoskeletal fitness of the abdominals, hamstrings, and back extensors work in concert to maintain posture and help maintain low back health.

Trunk Lift

Recommended

It is important that attention be given to performance technique during this test. The movement should be performed in a slow and controlled manner. The maximum score on this test is 12 inches. While some flexibility is important, it is not advisable (or safe) to encourage hyperextension.

Test Objective: To lift the upper body off the floor using the muscles of the back and hold the position to allow for the measurement.

Equipment/Facilities: Gym mats and a yardstick or 15 in. ruler are required to administer this test. It is helpful to mark the 6, 9 and 12 in. marks with colored tape.

Test Description: The student being tested lies on the mat in a prone position (face down). Toes are pointed and hands are placed under the thighs. Place a coin or other marker on the floor in line with the student's eyes. During the movement, the

MUSCLE STRENGTH, ENDURANCE, AND FLEXIBILITY

student's focus should not move from the coin or marker. The student lifts the upper body off the floor, in a very slow and controlled manner, to a maximum height of 12 in. (figures 4.15, 4.16, and 4.17). The position is held long enough to allow the tester to place the ruler on the floor in front of the student and determine the distance from the floor to the student's chin. The ruler should be placed at least an inch to the front of the student's chin and not directly under the chin. Once the measurement has been made the student returns to starting position in a controlled manner. Allow two trials, recording the highest score.

Scoring: The score is recorded to the nearest inch. Distances above 12 in. should be recorded as 12 in.

Suggestions for Test Administration:

• Do not allow students to do ballistic, bouncing movements.

• Do not encourage students to raise higher than 12 in. The Healthy Fitness Zone ends at 12 in., and scores beyond 12 in. will not be accepted by the computer. Excessive arching of the back may cause compression of the discs.

• Maintaining focus on the spot on the floor should assist in maintaining the head in a neutral position.

Upper Body Strength and Endurance

Strength and endurance of the muscles in the upper body are important in maintaining functional health and promoting good posture. The role of upper body strength in maintaining functionality becomes more evident as a person ages. It is important that children and youth learn the importance of upper body strength and endurance as well as methods to use in developing and maintaining this area of fitness. The 90° push-up is the recommended test item. Alternatives include the modified pull-up, pull-up, and flexed arm hang.

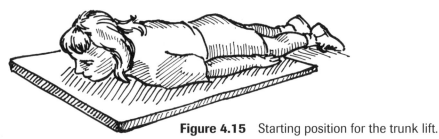

Figure 4.15 Starting position for the trunk lift.

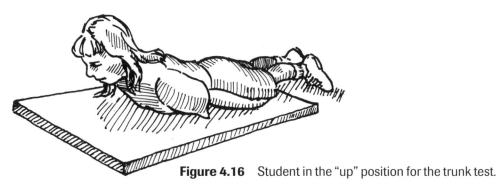

Figure 4.16 Student in the "up" position for the trunk test.

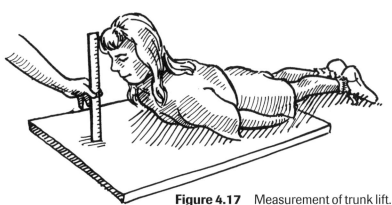

Figure 4.17 Measurement of trunk lift.

MUSCLE STRENGTH, ENDURANCE, AND FLEXIBILITY

Push-Up

Recommended

The push-up to an elbow angle of 90° is the recommended test for the upper body strength and endurance. Test administration requires little or no equipment, multiple students may be tested at one time, and few zero scores result. It also teaches students an activity that can be used throughout life as a conditioning activity as well as an item for use in self-testing.

Test Objective: To complete as many push-ups as possible at a rhythmic pace. This test item is used for males and females.

Equipment/Facilities: The only equipment necessary is an audio tape with the recorded cadence. The correct cadence is 20 push-ups per minute (1 push-up every 3 seconds). The PACER Test CD or tape contains a recorded push-up cadence.

Test Instructions: The students should be paired; one will perform the test while the other counts push-ups and watches to see that the student being tested bends the elbow to 90° with the upper arm parallel to the floor.

Prior to test day, students should be allowed to practice doing push-ups and watching their partner do them. Teachers should make a concerted effort during these practice sessions to correct students who are not achieving the 90° angle. In this manner all students will gain greater skill in knowing what 90° "feels like" and "looks like."

The student being tested assumes a prone position on the mat with hands placed under the shoulders, fingers stretched out, legs straight and slightly apart, and toes tucked under. The student pushes up off the mat with the arms until arms are straight, keeping legs and back straight. The back should be kept in a straight line from head to toes throughout the test (figure 4.18).

The student then lowers the body using the arms until the elbows bend at a 90° angle and the upper arms are parallel to the floor (figure 4.19). This movement is repeated as many times as possible. The student should continue the movement until the arms are straight each repetition. The rhythm should be approximately 20 push-ups per min or 1 push-up every 3 s.

When to Stop: Students are stopped when the second form correction is made.

Scoring: The score is the number of push-ups performed. For ease in administration, it is permissible to count the first incorrect push-up. It is important to be consistent with all of the students and classes.

Form Corrections:

- Stopping to rest or not maintaining a rhythmic pace
- Not achieving a 90° angle with the elbow on each repetition

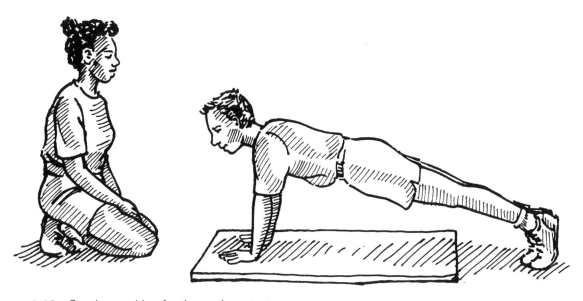

Figure 4.18   Starting position for the push-up test.

MUSCLE STRENGTH, ENDURANCE, AND FLEXIBILITY

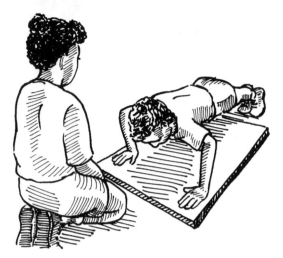

Figure 4.19 Student in the "down" position for the push-up test.

- Not maintaining correct body position
- Not extending arms fully

Suggestions for Test Administration:

- Test should be terminated if the student appears to be in extreme discomfort or pain.
- Cadence should be called or played on a prerecorded tape.
- Males and females follow the same protocol.

Modified Pull-Up

Alternative

For schools with access to equipment for the modified pull-up, it is a very good test item to use.

Test Objective: To successfully complete as many modified pull-ups as possible.

Equipment/Facilities: A modified pull-up stand, elastic band, pencil, and scoresheet are necessary to administer this test. See appendix A for instructions for constructing the modified pull-up stand.

Test Instructions: The student lies on her back with shoulders directly under a bar that has been set 1 to 2 inches above his reach. Place an elastic band 7 to 8 in. below and parallel to the bar.

The student grasps the bar with an overhand grip (palms away from body). The pull-up begins in "down" position with arms and legs straight, buttocks off the floor, and only the heels touching the floor. The student then pulls up until her chin is above the elastic band (figures 4.20 and 4.21).

When to Stop: Students are stopped when the second form correction is made.

Scoring: The score is the number of pull-ups performed. For ease in administration it is permissible to count the first incorrect pull-up. It is important to be consistent with all of the students and classes.

Suggestions for Test Administration:

- Movement should use only the arms. The body should be kept straight.

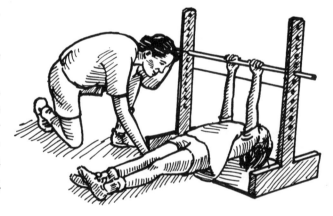

Figure 4.20 Starting position for the modified pull-up test.

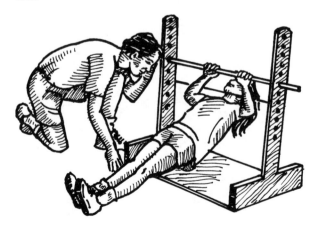

Figure 4.21 Student in the "up" position for the modified pull-up test.

MUSCLE STRENGTH, ENDURANCE, AND FLEXIBILITY

- Movement should be rhythmical and continuous. Students may not stop and rest.

- The test is terminated if the student experiences extreme discomfort or pain.

Pull-Up

Alternative

The pull-up test is not the recommended test item for the vast majority of students because many are unable to perform even one. This test item should not be used for students who cannot perform one repetition. However, for those students who are able to perform correct pull-ups it is a valid, reliable test option and is also an item that can be used throughout life as a conditioning activity as well as a self-test.

Test Objective: The object of this test is to correctly complete as many pull-ups as possible.

Equipment/Facilities: A horizontal bar at a height that allows the student to hang with arms fully extended and feet clear of the floor is used for this test. A doorway gym bar may be used.

Test Instructions: The student assumes a hanging position on the bar with an overhand grasp (palms facing away from the body) as illustrated in figure 4.22. Shorter students may be lifted into the starting position. The student uses her arms to pull her body up until her chin is above the bar (figure 4.23) and then lowers her body again into the full hanging position. The exercise is repeated as many times as possible. There is no time limit.

When to Stop: Students are stopped when the second form correction is made.

Scoring: The score is the number of complete pull-ups performed. For ease in administration, it is permissible to count the first incorrect pull-up. It is important to be consistent with all of the students and classes. The computer software will not accept a score of 0.

Form Corrections:

- The body should not swing during the movement. If the student starts to swing, the teacher or assistant should hold an arm in front of her thighs to prevent swinging.

- The pull-up must be performed smoothly with no kicking or jerking. Forceful bending of the knees is not permitted.

- To be counted, a pull-up must result in the chin's being lifted over the bar and the student must return to the full hanging position with elbows fully extended.

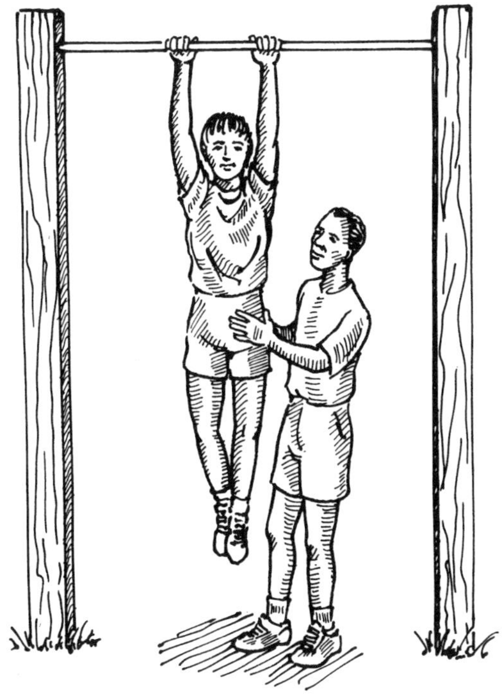

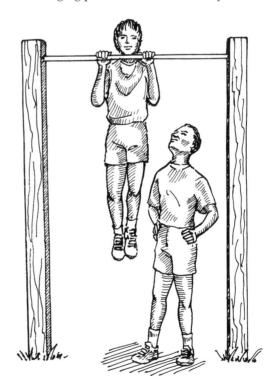

Figure 4.23   Student in the "up" position for the pull-up test.

Figure 4.22   Starting position for the pull-up test.

MUSCLE STRENGTH, ENDURANCE, AND FLEXIBILITY

Flexed Arm Hang
Alternative

Test Objective: The objective of the flexed arm hang is to hang with the chin above the bar as long as possible.

Equipment/Facilities: A horizontal bar, chair, and stopwatch are required to administer this test item.

Test Instructions: The student grasps the bar with an overhand grip (palms facing away). With the assistance of one or more spotters, the student raises his body off the floor to a position where his chin is above the bar, elbows are flexed, and chest is close to the bar (figures 4.24 and 4.25). A stopwatch is started as soon as the student takes this position. The position is held as long as possible. The watch is stopped when one of the following occurs: the student's chin touches the bar, his head tilts backward to keep his chin above the bar, or his chin falls below the level of the bar.

When to Stop: Students are stopped when the chin drops below the bar or when the second form correction is made.

Scoring: The score is the number of seconds the student is able to maintain the correct hanging position.

Suggestions for Test Administration:

• The body must not swing during the test. If the student starts to swing, the teacher or assistant should hold an extended arm across the front of the thighs to prevent the swinging motion.

• Only one trial is permitted unless the teacher believes that the pupil has not had a fair opportunity to perform.

Flexibility

Maintaining adequate joint flexibility is important to functional health. However, for young people decreased flexibility is generally not a problem. Many of your students will easily pass the flexibility item; therefore, the flexibility item has been made optional. If you decide not to administer the flexibility test, remember you should teach students about flexibility and inform them that maintaining flexibility and range of motion will be important as they age.

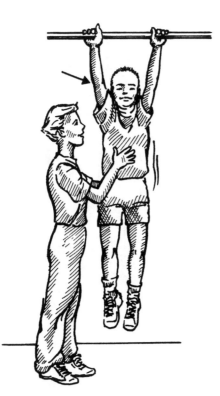

Figure 4.24 Starting position for the flexed arm hang test.

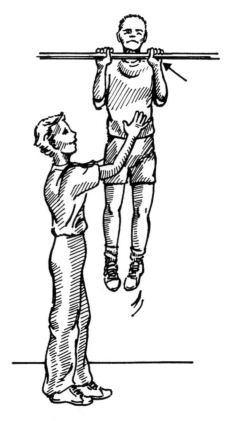

Figure 4.25 Student in the "up" position for the flexed arm hang test.

MUSCLE STRENGTH, ENDURANCE, AND FLEXIBILITY

Back-Saver Sit and Reach

Optional

The back-saver sit and reach is very similar to the traditional sit and reach except that the measurement is performed on one side at a time. This is so that students are not encouraged to hyperextend. The sit and reach measures predominantly the flexibility of the hamstring muscles. Normal hamstring flexibility allows rotation of the pelvis in forward bending movements and posterior tilting of the pelvis for proper sitting.

Test Objective: To be able to reach the specified distance on the right and left sides of the body. The distance required to achieve Healthy Fitness Zone is adjusted for age and gender and is specified in tables 5.1 and 5.2 on pages 38 and 39.

Equipment/Facilities: This assessment requires a sturdy box approximately 12 inches high. A measuring scale is placed on top of the box with the 9 in. mark parallel to the face of the box against which the student's foot will rest. The "zero" end of the ruler is nearest the student. Instructions for construction of a special measuring apparatus are contained in appendix A. However, a wooden box and yardstick will suffice.

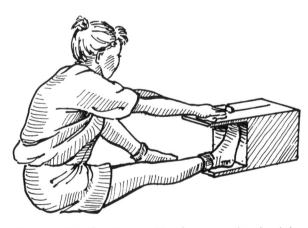

Figure 4.26 Starting position for measuring the right side.

Test Description: The student removes her shoes and sits down at the test apparatus. One leg is fully extended with the foot flat against the face of the box. The other knee is bent with the sole of the foot flat on the floor and 2-3 inches to the side of the straight knee. The arms are extended forward over the measuring scale with the hands placed one on top of the other (figure 4.26). With palms down, the student reaches directly forward with both hands along the scale four times and holds the position of the fourth reach for at least 1 second (figure 4.27). After measuring one side the student switches the position of the legs and reaches again. The student may allow the bent knee to move to the side as the body moves by it if necessary.

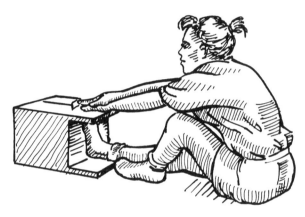

Fig. 4.27 Back-saver sit and reach stretch for the right side.

Scoring: Record the number of inches on each side to the nearest half inch reached to a maximum score of 12 in. Performance is limited to discourage hypermobility.

Suggestions for Test Administration:

• The bent knee moves to the side allowing the body to move past it.

• The knee of the extended leg should remain straight. Tester may place one hand on the student's knee to remind her to keep the knee straight.

• Hands should reach forward evenly.

• The trial should be repeated if the hands reach unevenly or the knee bends.

• Hips must remain square to the box. Do not allow the student to turn the hip away from the box as she reaches.

MUSCLE STRENGTH, ENDURANCE, AND FLEXIBILITY

Shoulder Stretch

Optional

The shoulder stretch is a simple test of upper body flexibility. If used alternately with the back saver sit and reach, it may be useful in educating students that flexibility is important in all areas of the body, not just the hamstring muscles.

Test Objective: To be able to touch the fingertips together behind the back by reaching over the shoulder and under the elbow.

Equipment/Facilities: No equipment is necessary to complete this test item.

Test Description: Allow students to select a partner. The partner judges ability to complete the stretch.

To test the right shoulder, the student reaches with her right hand over her right shoulder and down the back as if to pull up a zipper. At the same time she places her left hand behind her back and

reaches up, trying to touch the fingers of the right hand (figure 4.28). Her partner observes whether the fingers touch.

To test the left shoulder, the student reaches with her left hand over his left shoulder and down the back as if to pull up a zipper. At the same time she places his right hand behind his back and reaches up, trying to touch the fingers of the left hand (figure 4.29). Her partner notes whether her fingers touch.

Scoring: If the student is able to touch her fingers with her right hand over her shoulder, a "Y" is recorded for the right side; if not, an "N" is recorded. If the student is able to touch her fingers with her left hand over the shoulder, a "Y" is recorded for the left side; otherwise an "N" is recorded.

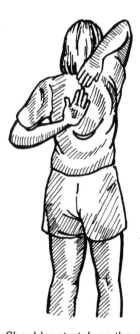

Figure 4.28 Shoulder stretch on the right side.

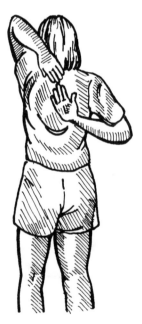

Figure 4.29 Shoulder stretch on the left side.

FITNESSGRAM PHYSICAL ACTIVITY QUESTIONNAIRE

The Physical Activity Questionnaire was added to the children's version of the *FITNESSGRAM* software to improve the prescriptive information that is given to the child. Many factors, including heredity, maturation, and body composition, can influence a child's performance on physical fitness tests. Some children may get discouraged if they do not score well on fitness tests despite being active. Alternately, other children may incorrectly believe that they don't need to be active if their fitness levels are adequate. The activity assessment will allow for more personalized and prescriptive information on the *FITNESSGRAM* report. This feedback will reinforce the notion that it is important to be physically active regardless of fitness level.

Description

The assessment includes three brief questions that are based on items from the Youth Risk Behavior Survey—a national surveillance instrument used to track nationwide trends in physical activity. Each question asks the students to report the number of days in a given week in which they performed different forms of physical activity (aerobic, strength, and flexibility). The wording of the questions is provided below:

Aerobic Activity Question

On how many of the past 7 days did you participate in physical activity for a total of 30-60 minutes or more over the course of a day? This includes moderate activities (walking, slow bicycling, or outdoor play) as well as vigorous activities (jogging, active games, or active sports such as basketball, tennis, or soccer). (0, 1, 2, 3, 4, 5, 6, 7 days)

Strength Activity Question

On how many of the past 7 days did you do exercises to strengthen your muscles? This includes exercises such as push-ups, sit-ups, or weight lifting. (0, 1, 2, 3, 4, 5, 6, 7 days)

Flexibility Activity Question

On how many of the past 7 days did you do stretching exercises to loosen up or relax your muscles? This includes exercises such as toe touches, knee bending, or leg stretching. (0, 1, 2, 3, 4, 5, 6, 7 days)

Administration

Because it may be difficult for young children to accurately recall this information, the activity assessments may not be valid for children from grades K-4. To increase the validity of this assessment it is recommended that teachers prepare the students to answer these questions ahead of time. Be sure to explain the different types of physical activity (aerobic, strength, and flexibility) and illustrate (with examples) how to count the number of days of activity. This could be done as part of an effort to teach children about how much physical activity they should try to do each week. Physical activity guidelines used in *FITNESSGRAM* and *ACTIVITYGRAM* software are outlined in appendix B.

Chapter 5 | Interpreting *FITNESSGRAM* Results

FITNESSGRAM uses criterion-referenced standards to evaluate fitness performance. These standards have been established to represent a level of fitness that offers some degree of protection against diseases, which result from sedentary living. Performance is classified in two general areas: "Needs Improvement" and "Healthy Fitness Zone" (HFZ). Tables 5.1 and 5.2 provide a list of standards for the HFZ. All students should strive to achieve a score that places them inside the HFZ. It is possible for some students to score above the HFZ. *FITNESSGRAM* acknowledges performances above the HFZ but does not recommend this level of performance as an appropriate goal level for all students. However, students who desire to achieve a high level of athletic performance may need to consider setting goals beyond the HFZ. Students, especially younger students, may need assistance in setting realistic goals.

Healthy Fitness Zone

Needs Improvement	Good	Better

Remember, when administering *FITNESSGRAM* test items to students in grades K-3, performance level is not the most important objective. Children in this group should focus more on learning to perform the test items successfully.

Research findings were used as the basis for establishing the *FITNESSGRAM* health fitness standards. With regard to aerobic fitness level, Blair et al. (1989) reported that a significant decrease in risk of all-cause mortality results from getting out of the lower 20% of the population. They also reported that risk level continues to decrease as fitness levels increase, but not as dramatically as simply getting out of the bottom 20%. Aerobic capacity standards for the HFZ have been established so that the lower end of the Healthy Fitness Zone corresponds closely to a fitness level equal to getting out of the lower 20% of the population. The upper end of the Healthy Fitness Zone corresponds to a fitness level that would include up to 60% of the population.

Percentage fat is calculated from equations reported by Slaughter et al. (1988). Detailed information on the development of these equations and other issues related to the measurement and interpretation of body composition information is available in *Advances in Body Composition Assessment* (Lohman 1992). Williams et al. (1992) reported that children with body fat levels above 25% for boys and 30 to 35% for girls are more likely to exhibit elevated cholesterol levels and hypertension. The beginning of the HFZ corresponds to these levels of body fatness.

Little or no data exist to indicate levels of musculoskeletal fitness associated with good health. Standards in this area of fitness were established to correspond in level as closely as possible to those in aerobic capacity and body composition.

In interpreting performance on physical fitness assessments, it is most important to remember the following:

- The physical fitness experience should always be fun and enjoyable.
- Physical fitness testing should not become a competitive sport.
- The performance of one student should not be compared to that of another student.
- The primary reason for testing is to provide the student with personal information that may be used in planning a personal fitness program.
- The performance level on fitness tests should not be used as a basis for grading.

Influence of Body Size and Maturity on Fitness

Body size (height and weight) is to some extent related to physical fitness as measured by a combination of tests. Although there is much variability among individuals, the influence of body size on fitness is especially apparent in two ways:

1. Excess weight associated with fatness tends to have a negative influence on aerobic capacity and on test items in which the body must be lifted or moved (e.g., upper body strength items).

2. Variation in body size associated with maturity can influence fitness around the time of the adolescent growth spurt and sexual maturation. There is considerable variation among individuals

in the timing of this maturation period. In adequately nourished children, the timing is largely determined by genetics. Within a given age group of early adolescent children, there will be great variation in the maturation level.

This variation in size will influence performance on fitness tests. Boys show a clear growth spurt in muscle mass, strength, power, and endurance and a decrease in subcutaneous fat on the arms and legs. Girls show considerably smaller growth spurts in strength, power, and endurance and tend to accumulate body fat compared to boys. In this age-group children may experience an increase or decrease in their abilities to perform on certain test items completely independent of their levels of physical activity.

In addition to being influenced by maturity a child's response to training is also determined by genetic background. Some children will improve performance more rapidly than others. Some children will be able to perform at a much higher level than others regardless of training levels.

Features of the *FITNESSGRAM* Report

The *FITNESSGRAM* has numerous special features as illustrated in figure 5.1:

1. Generates highly personalized output.
2. Indicates current and past test performance.
3. Makes individualized recommendations based on assessment results.
4. Recommendations and feedback.
5. Evaluates performance based on criterion-referenced health standards. Classifies scores in the Needs Improvement area, the Healthy Fitness Zone, or above the Healthy Fitness Zone.
6. Includes a bar graph of current and past assessment results.
7. Provides an estimated $\dot{V}O_2$max adjusted according to kilograms of body weight per minute that will allow comparison between performances on alternative test items.
8. Reports changes in height and weight.

Aerobic Capacity

Aerobic capacity indicates the ability of the respiratory, cardiovascular, and muscular systems to take up, transport, and utilize oxygen during exercise

FITNESSGRAM®

	Test Date	Height	Weight
Current	07/15/99	5'01"	105
Past	07/13/99	5'3"	122

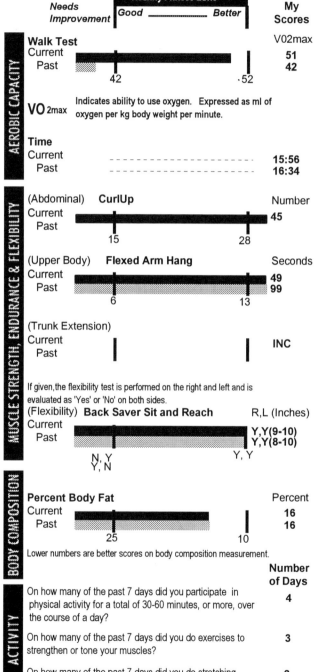

AEROBIC CAPACITY

	Healthy Fitness Zone	My Scores
	Needs Improvement / Good — Better	

Walk Test

VO2max
- Current: 51
- Past: 42

(scale: 42 ... -52)

VO 2max Indicates ability to use oxygen. Expressed as ml of oxygen per kg body weight per minute.

Time
- Current: 15:56
- Past: 16:34

MUSCLE STRENGTH, ENDURANCE & FLEXIBILITY

(Abdominal) CurlUp — Number
- Current: 45
- Past:

(scale: 15 ... 28)

(Upper Body) Flexed Arm Hang — Seconds
- Current: 49
- Past: 99

(scale: 6 ... 13)

(Trunk Extension)
- Current: INC
- Past:

If given, the flexibility test is performed on the right and left and is evaluated as 'Yes' or 'No' on both sides.

(Flexibility) Back Saver Sit and Reach — R,L (Inches)
- Current: Y,Y(9-10)
- Past: Y,Y(8-10)

N, Y
Y, N   Y, Y

BODY COMPOSITION

Percent Body Fat — Percent
- Current: 16
- Past: 16

(scale: 25 ... 10)

Lower numbers are better scores on body composition measurement.

ACTIVITY

	Number of Days
On how many of the past 7 days did you participate in physical activity for a total of 30-60 minutes, or more, over the course of a day?	4
On how many of the past 7 days did you do exercises to strengthen or tone your muscles?	3
On how many of the past 7 days did you do stretching exercises to loosen up or relax your muscles?	2

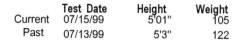

MESSAGES

Charlie, your scores on all test items were in or above the Healthy Fitness Zone. You are also doing strength and flexibility exercises. However, you need to play active games, sports or other activities at least 5 days each week.

Although your aerobic capacity score is in the Healthy Fitness Zone now, you are not doing enough physical activity. You should try to play very actively at least 60 minutes at least five days each week to look and feel good.

Your abdominal strength was very good. To maintain your fitness level be sure that your strength activities include curl-ups 3 to 5 days each week. Remember to keep your knees bent. Avoid having someone hold your feet.

Your upper body strength was very good, Charlie. To maintain your fitness level be sure that your strength activities include arm exercises such as push-ups, modified push-ups or climbing activities 2 to 3 days each week.

Charlie, your flexibility is in the Healthy Fitness Zone. To maintain your fitness, stretch slowly 3 or 4 days each week, holding the stretch 20 - 30 seconds. Don't forget that you need to stretch all areas of the body.

Charlie, your body composition is in the Healthy Fitness Zone. If you will be active most days each week, it may help to maintain your level of body composition.

To be healthy and fit it is important to do some physical activity almost every day. Aerobic exercise is good for your heart and body composition. Strength and flexibilty exercises are good for your muscles and joints.

Good job, you are doing enough physical activity for your health. Additional vigorous activity would help to promote higher levels of fitness.

©The Cooper Institute for Aerobics Research

Figure 5.1 Sample *FITNESSGRAM* computer report.

and activity. A laboratory measure of $\dot{V}O_2$max is generally the best measure of aerobic capacity. In addition to providing the actual score on the one-mile run/walk, the Pacer, or the walk test, *FITNESSGRAM* calculates an estimated $\dot{V}O_2$max that may be used to compare performance from one test date to another on the two different test items.

A low score on the field test estimates of aerobic capacity may be influenced by many factors. These include:

- actual aerobic capacity level,
- body composition,
- running and walking efficiency and economy,
- motivation level during the actual testing experience,
- extreme environmental conditions,
- ability to pace on the one-mile run and the walk test, and
- innate ability.

Improvement in any of these factors may improve the test score.

Aerobic capacity can be improved substantially in an unconditioned person who participates regularly in sustained activities involving large muscle groups. The amount of improvement is related to the beginning level of fitness and to the intensity, duration, and frequency of the training. The major part of the improvement will occur during the first six months. Thereafter, improvement will be much slower. Boys and girls who are overfat may expect an improvement in the aerobic capacity measure with a reduction in body fat.

For boys, aerobic capacity relative to body weight stays relatively constant during the growing years. For girls, aerobic capacity tends to remain constant between ages 5 and 10 years but decreases after age 10 due to increasing sex-specific essential fat.

One-mile run and PACER test scores tend to improve progressively with age in boys even though $\dot{V}O_2$max expressed relative to body weight tends to remain constant, because running economy improves. In 10- to 12-year-old girls, these field test scores also tend to improve due to improved running economy, but between ages 12 and 18, scores tend to remain relatively constant because improved running economy is offset by declining $\dot{V}O_2$max expressed relative to body weight. The differences in age-related changes in the relation of the one-mile run or PACER test scores to running economy are taken into account when the scores are converted to estimate $\dot{V}O_2$max by equations in the *FITNESSGRAM* program software.

Body Composition

Body composition standards have been established for both percent body fat calculated from triceps and calf skinfold measurements (for college students abdominal skinfold is also included) and body mass index calculated from measurements of weight and height. The standards represent the boundaries of the HFZ. Scores that fall either below or above this zone should receive attention for these students have greater potential to develop health problems related to their level of fatness or leanness.

Tables 5.3 and 5.4 have been adapted to indicate the HFZ for both percent fat and body mass index. The HFZ begins at 25% fat for the boys (20 to 27.8 BMI depending on age) and 32% fat for girls (21 to 27.3 BMI depending on age). Please notice that there is an optimal range within the HFZ. Ideally students should strive to be within this optimal range, which is 10 to 20% fat for boys and 15 to 25% fat for girls. Using this chart may simplify the explanation of the body composition assessment item. A body mass index in the "Needs Improvement" range indicates that the student's weight is too heavy for the height.

When interpreting body composition scores, it is important to remember the following:

- Skinfold measurements offer an estimate of body fatness.
- A 3 to 5% body fat measurement error is associated with the skinfold method.
- Body mass index provides an estimate of the appropriateness of the weight for the height.
- Body mass index may falsely identify a very muscular lean person as being overfat (too heavy for height) or a lightweight person with little muscular development and a large percent fat as being in the HFZ when they are actually overfat.

In general, students who score in the area below the HFZ should be encouraged to work toward this area by slowly changing their body weight through increased physical activity and decreased consumption of high-fat, high-calorie, low-nutrition foods. Changing dietary habits and exercise habits can be most difficult. Students with severe obesity or eating disorders may need professional assistance in their attempts to modify these aspects of their lifestyle. We cannot emphasize enough that health risks from obesity are greatly reduced if the child is physically active.

It is important to remember in interpreting body composition results that most students who are overfat may also have performances in other test areas that are outside the HFZ. An improvement in body composition will generally result in an improved performance in aerobic capacity and also muscle strength and endurance, especially in the upper body, due to a reduction in excess weight.

For children above the age of twelve years, the *FITNESSGRAM* also identifies students who are very lean, having less than 8% fat for boys (less than 13.1 to 17.0 BMI depending on age) and 13% fat for girls (less than 14.1 to 15.0 BMI depending upon age) with a message indicating that being this lean may not be best for health. Parents and teachers should notice students who are categorized as being very lean and consider factors that may be responsible for their low level of body fat. Many students may naturally be very lean while others may have inappropriate nutritional patterns. A few students may be suffering from an eating disorder. A factor to consider is whether the student's level of fat has suddenly changed from within the optimal range to a level identified as very lean. Severe changes may signal a potential problem. Creating awareness of a child's current status is the primary purpose in identifying lean students. Changes in status should be monitored.

FITNESSGRAM results can be very helpful in allowing students to follow changes in their levels of body fat over time. Obesity is a health problem both for children and adults. Childhood is the most appropriate time to address problems or potential problems and attempt to make the necessary behavior change to remedy problems in this area of health-related fitness. Long-term effects on reducing body fat in children have been shown to occur by educating children and their parents about body composition, physical activity, and diet (Epstein et al. 1990).

Muscle Strength, Endurance, and Flexibility

Students who score poorly in one or more areas of muscle strength, endurance, and flexibility should be encouraged to participate in calisthenics and other strengthening and stretching activities that will develop those areas. However, it is essential to remember that physical fitness training is very specific and the areas of the body being tested represent only a fraction of the total body.

To focus on activities which develop the extensors of the arms without equal attention to the flexors of the arms will not accomplish the important objective, which is to develop an overall healthy musculoskeletal system. Remember, you must have strength and flexibility in the muscles on both sides of every joint. A useful activity for all students is to identify exercises to strengthen and stretch the muscles at every major joint of the trunk, upper body, and lower body.

Poor performance on the measures of abdominal strength and trunk extensor strength and flexibility may merit special attention. Gaining strength and flexibility in these areas may help prevent low back pain, which affects millions of people, young and old.

Physical Activity Questionnaire

If the Physical Activity Questionnaire is completed, the individualized feedback provided on the *FITNESSGRAM* report will factor in the child's responses to the physical activity questions. If children do not complete the questions, then the feedback will be based only on their fitness scores. The conceptual matrix in table 5.5 illustrates the general content of the integrated fitness and activity feedback. The actual feedback will be specific for each dimension of fitness (aerobic, musculoskeletal, and body composition) and will be more detailed, but this chart illustrates the general concept.

Recognition

FITNESSGRAM does not advocate a recognition program that focuses primarily on fitness performance. Recognition should reinforce the establishment of activity behaviors that will lead to fitness development. *You Stay Active!* (see chapter 9) is the recommended recognition program. A part of *You Stay Active!* is a goal-setting recognition system that can be used to acknowledge individual performance level based on personal goals.

Table 5.1 *FITNESSGRAM* Standards for Healthy Fitness Zone*

BOYS

Age	One-mile run (min:sec)		PACER (# laps)		Walk test & $\dot{V}O_2$max (ml/kg/min)		Percent fat		Body mass index		Curl-up (# complete)	
5	Completion of distance. Time standards not recommended.		Participation in run. Lap count standards not recommended.				25	10	20	14.7	2	10
6							25	10	20	14.7	2	10
7							25	10	20	14.9	4	14
8							25	10	20	15.1	6	20
9							25	10	20	15.2	9	24
10	11:30	9:00	23	61	42	52	25	10	21	15.3	12	24
11	11:00	8:30	23	72	42	52	25	10	21	15.8	15	28
12	10:30	8:00	32	72	42	52	25	10	22	16.0	18	36
13	10:00	7:30	41	72	42	52	25	10	23	16.6	21	40
14	9:30	7:00	41	83	42	52	25	10	24.5	17.5	24	45
15	9:00	7:00	51	94	42	52	25	10	25	18.1	24	47
16	8:30	7:00	61	94	42	52	25	10	26.5	18.5	24	47
17	8:30	7:00	61	94	42	52	25	10	27	18.8	24	47
17+	8:30	7:00	61	94	42	52	25	10	27.8	19.0	24	47

Age	Trunk lift (inches)		Push-up (# complete)		Modified pull-up (# complete)		Pull-up (# complete)		Flexed arm hang (seconds)		Back-saver sit & reach** (inches)	Shoulder stretch
5	6	12	3	8	2	7	1	2	2	8	8	
6	6	12	3	8	2	7	1	2	2	8	8	
7	6	12	4	10	3	9	1	2	3	8	8	
8	6	12	5	13	4	11	1	2	3	8	8	Passing = touching fingertips together behind the back
9	6	12	6	15	5	11	1	2	4	10	8	
10	9	12	7	20	5	15	1	2	4	10	8	
11	9	12	8	20	6	17	1	3	6	13	8	
12	9	12	10	20	7	20	1	3	6	13	8	
13	9	12	12	25	8	22	1	4	12	17	8	
14	9	12	14	30	9	25	2	5	15	20	8	
15	9	12	16	35	10	27	3	7	15	20	8	
16	9	12	18	35	12	30	5	8	15	20	8	
17	9	12	18	35	14	30	5	8	15	20	8	
17+	9	12	18	35	14	30	5	8	15	20	8	

* Number on left is lower end of HFZ; number on right is upper end of HFZ

**Test scored Pass/Fail; must reach this distance to pass.

©1992, 1999, The Cooper Institute for Aerobics Research, Dallas, Texas.

Table 5.2 *FITNESSGRAM* Standards for Healthy Fitness Zone*

GIRLS

Age	One-mile run min:sec		PACER # laps		Walk test & V̇O₂max ml/kg/min		Percent fat		Body mass index		Curl-up # complete	
5	Completion of distance. Time standards not recommended.		Participation in run. Lap count standards not recommended.				32	17	21	16.2	2	10
6							32	17	21	16.2	2	10
7							32	17	22	16.2	4	14
8							32	17	22	16.2	6	20
9							32	17	23	16.2	9	22
10	12:30	9:30	15	41	40	48	32	17	23.5	16.6	12	26
11	12:00	9:00	15	41	39	47	32	17	24	16.9	15	29
12	12:00	9:00	23	41	38	46	32	17	24.5	16.9	18	32
13	11:30	9:00	23	51	37	45	32	17	24.5	17.5	18	32
14	11:00	8:30	23	51	36	44	32	17	25	17.5	18	32
15	10:30	8:00	23	51	35	43	32	17	25	17.5	18	35
16	10:00	8:00	32	61	35	43	32	17	25	17.5	18	35
17	10:00	8:00	41	61	35	43	32	17	26	17.5	18	35
17+	10:00	8:00	41	61	35	43	32	17	27.3	18.0	18	35

Age	Trunk lift inches		Push-up # complete		Modified pull-up # complete		Pull-up # complete		Flexed arm hang seconds		Back-saver sit & reach** inches	Shoulder stretch
5	6	12	3	8	2	7	1	2	2	8	9	
6	6	12	3	8	2	7	1	2	2	8	9	
7	6	12	4	10	3	9	1	2	3	8	9	
8	6	12	5	13	4	11	1	2	3	10	9	
9	6	12	6	15	4	11	1	2	4	10	9	Passing = touching fingertips together behind the back
10	9	12	7	15	4	13	1	2	4	10	9	
11	9	12	7	15	4	13	1	2	6	12	10	
12	9	12	7	15	4	13	1	2	7	12	10	
13	9	12	7	15	4	13	1	2	8	12	10	
14	9	12	7	15	4	13	1	2	8	12	10	
15	9	12	7	15	4	13	1	2	8	12	12	
16	9	12	7	15	4	13	1	2	8	12	12	
17	9	12	7	15	4	13	1	2	8	12	12	
17+	9	12	7	15	4	13	1	2	8	12	12	

* Number on left is lower end of HFZ; number on right is upper end of HFZ

**Test scored Pass/Fail; must reach this distance to pass.

©1992, 1999, The Cooper Institute for Aerobics Research, Dallas, Texas.

Table 5.3 The *FITNESSGRAM* Body Composition Classification

BOYS

Percent fat (All ages)	42	38	35	31	28	24 (25)	20	17	13	10	7
	Very high				High	Mod. high	Optimal range			Low	Very low
	Needs improvement					Healthy Fitness Zone					Lean message

Body mass index (Age)			
5	20	14.7	
6	20	14.7	
7	20	14.9	
8	20	15.1	
9	20	15.2	
10	21	15.3	
11	21	15.8	
12	22	16.0	
13	23	16.6	15.0
14	24.5	17.5	15.7
15	25	18.1	16.4
16	26.5	18.5	16.6
17	27	18.8	16.8
18-25	27.8	19.0	17.0

Adapted, by permission, from T. Lohman, 1987, "The use of skinfold to estimate body fatness in children and youth," *Journal of Physical Education, Recreation and Dance* 58: 98-102.

Table 5.4   The *FITNESSGRAM* Body Composition Classification

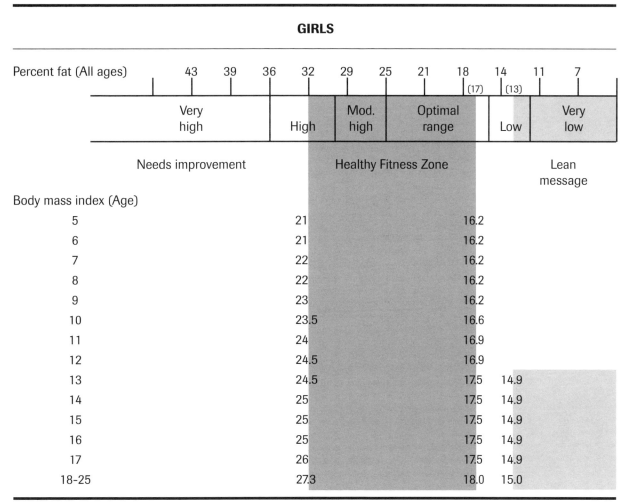

Adapted, by permission, from T. Lohman, 1987, "The use of skinfold to estimate body fatness in children and youth," *Journal of Physical Education, Recreation and Dance* 58: 98-102.

Table 5.5   Conceptual Matrix Used to Integrate Fitness and Activity Results

	Physically Active?	
Fitness Results	**Yes**	**No**
Scores in Healthy Fitness Zone	Congratulations, you are in the Healthy Fitness Zone. You are doing regular physical activity and this is keeping you fit.	Congratulations, you are in the Healthy Fitness Zone. To keep fit it is important that you do regular physical activity.
Scores not in Healthy Fitness Zone	Even though your scores are not in the Healthy Fitness Zone, you are doing enough physical activity. Keep up the good work.	Your scores were not in the Healthy Fitness Zone. Try to increase your activity levels to improve your fitness and health.

Chapter 6 | Modification of *FITNESSGRAM* for Special Populations

Other sections of this manual present *FITNESSGRAM* as intended for use with students who are not disabled. You will, in many situations, also be working with students who possess disabilities. If certain physical fitness components are deemed important as a dimension in education, they are equally important for all students. General and specific suggestions are provided for modifying testing procedures, the *FITNESSGRAM* report, and the recognition program so that the physical fitness needs of the student with disabilities can be fully addressed.

Specific criterion standards for students with disabilities are not available. The activities described within this section may be used to establish an individual baseline for each student. Performances on subsequent assessments can be compared to this baseline performance. You can also use the baseline data as a guideline in establishing individual goals, which may be used as a "standard" for the individual. Essentially, it is possible to use any task as the assessment by establishing a baseline and comparing progress back to that baseline performance. Teachers needing assistance in developing tasks for an assessment should consult one of these excellent resources: *Physical Fitness Testing of the Disabled: Project Unique* (Winnick and Short 1985) and *Physical Best and Children with Disabilities* (AAHPERD 1996).

Test Administration

Until recently, many students with disabilities were simply exempted from physical fitness assessment and developmental activities. As a result, many of these students are not familiar with physical fitness assessment techniques. You will have to teach students how to take the fitness test items. Valid and reliable measures of physical fitness components can never be obtained if the student fails to understand how to take the test.

On days preceding the assessment, it is appropriate for students to practice the test items. If, for any reason, you suspect that the student with disabilities does not understand the administration of a test, you should provide instruction and a chance to practice. Of special concern is ensuring that the student understands the verbal instructions. Verbal descriptions presented to students with disabilities are often interpreted differently than when presented to the nondisabled. This is due to differences in previous movement or motor learning experiences. As students with disabilities become familiar with the specific procedures of the physical fitness test items, and as the fitness status of these students is assessed at regular intervals, the need for practice time will diminish.

Aerobic Capacity

The aerobic capacity test presents two problems for students with disabilities. First, some students are simply not able to run. For those students, a running test is not appropriate. Conditions that may preclude running include those requiring a wheelchair, braces, or other assistive devices for mobility, leg amputation, congenital anomalies, arthritis, and some vision impairments. Second, some students cannot safely participate in a maximal or near maximal test of the functional status of the cardiorespiratory system. Acute asthma, cystic fibrosis, and some congenital coronary conditions would be examples of conditions under which maximal tests should not be used. For these students, a submaximal assessment should be completed.

In cases where the student is unable to run, there are a number of alternatives. In maximal aerobic capacity assessments, the objective is to have a large muscle mass completing moderate to heavy exercise for an extended period of time. The mode of exercise is not particularly important as long as a large muscle mass is involved. Swimming, stationary bicycling using the arms or the legs to pedal, propelling a wheelchair, and walking are examples of exercise that require a large muscle mass. Although standards for these activities are unavailable, improvements in performance subsequent to conditioning may be accepted as probable improvements in aerobic capacity.

Swimming

If you elect to use swimming as the mode of exercise, the student should possess swimming skill or may use a flotation device. However, you should see that the student uses the same flotation device in all subsequent assessments. The distance of the swim should be 300 yards for younger elementary students, 400 yards for upper elementary students, 500 yards for junior high students, and 700 yards for high school students. The score on the test is the time taken to complete the distance. Standards are unavailable, but improvements in time subsequent to conditioning are accepted as improvements in aerobic capacity.

Stationary Bicycle

In using the stationary bicycle, pedaling may be done with the arms or the legs. The stationary bicycle used must be constructed so that exact workload or distance covered can be determined. With the resistance set at a moderate level, the student makes as many pedal revolutions as possible in 5 minutes. The number of pedal revolutions or the distance covered during the 5 min period is the score for the test. The resistance should remain constant in subsequent testing sessions.

Propelling a Wheelchair

If the student is propelling a wheelchair, the goal is to cover a specific distance in the minimal amount of time. For younger elementary students, the distance should be 600 yards; older elementary students should use 800 yd, junior high students 1,200 yd, and high school students 1 mi. When assessment is repeated, you should make certain the student uses the same wheelchair and the same facility. Changes in the wheelchair or the testing surface will make comparisons to previous times invalid. The score is the time required to cover the distance.

Walking

In walking, younger elementary students should walk 600 yards, older elementary students should walk 800 yd, junior high students should walk 1,200 yd, and high school students should walk 1 mi. Near maximal exercise is approximated if the distance is covered in the minimal amount of time possible.

The recommendations presented above are for students with disabilities whose condition allows for maximal or near-maximal estimates of aerobic capacity. The distances are arbitrary selections and may be modified based on individual capabilities. The results of the assessment are not comparable to performances on the one-mile run/walk. The assessment is, however, important to the student with disabilities because when the assessment is repeated, improvement in performance is probably due to an improvement in aerobic capacity. If, on the other hand, there is considerable deterioration in the performance during the subsequent assessment, the deterioration may be due to a decrease in aerobic capacity.

If a student has a disability whereby a maximal or near-maximal effort puts the student at risk, the criteria for selecting the intensity of the exercise must be modified. For students at risk, the recommended modification is to change the rate of work so that the student uses a large muscle mass to work at a mild rate for an extended period of time. In this case, the heart rate during exercise should not exceed 120 beats per min. Stationary bicycling, walking, running, or swimming may be used as the mode of exercise. You select a pace that will maintain the student's heart rate below 120 beats per minute, and the student completes the exercise period as indicated above for those not at risk. During the first 10 to 15 s post-exercise, you monitor the student's heart rate. During subsequent assessments, if the student covers the same distance in the same period of time and the monitored heart rate is lower, this may be taken as an indication that the aerobic capacity has probably improved. An increase in the monitored heart rate may be an indication of a deterioration in aerobic capacity.

Body Composition

The *FITNESSGRAM* field assessment for body fatness utilizes the triceps and calf skinfold thicknesses. Skinfold measurements of subcutaneous fat on students with scar tissue at these locations should not be used to estimate body fat. Nor should you take skinfold measurements at sites where students receive repeated subdural and/or intramuscular injections. Limbs that have muscle atrophy should not be used.

The procedures outlined for body composition in this manual indicate that all skinfold measurements should be made on the right side of the body. If problems preclude measurement of skinfold thicknesses on the right side of the body, then it is permissible to take measurements on the left side. In some cases, it may be necessary to mix measurements from both the right and left sides of the body. The mixing of measurements from the two sides of the body is preferable to no measurement or to the measurement of a single site. If only a single site can be measured, the norms presented in Johnston et al. (1972, 1974) may be used. If, on the other hand, none of the sites can be measured, you should measure a vertical skinfold on the abdomen 2 in. to the right of the umbilicus. This measurement would not be comparable to the sites used in *FITNESSGRAM* but it can serve as a reference point for the student for future measurements. If this skinfold increases over time, the student probably has an increase in total body fat. A decrease in this measure may indicate a decrease in total body fat.

Muscle Strength, Endurance, and Flexibility

Virtually any movement may be used as a test of muscular strength and flexibility. Students may be asked to do the movement as many times as they can with or without a time limit or to do a certain number of repetitions. Students with motor control problems will probably need to have any timing factors removed from the assessment as long as the movement is rhythmic and the student does not pause longer than 2 s between repetitions. Some students may need more warm-up prior to attempting a flexibility test. The important consideration is to establish a baseline performance which may be used as a basis of comparison to determine progress in strength development.

Modification of the *FITNESSGRAM* Report

The *FITNESSGRAM* computer software is programmed with standards established for the student who is not disabled. Although the standards compare the student's performance to a health-referenced standard rather than to the performance of other students, the use of these standards to evaluate the performance of a student with disabilities may not be appropriate. The *FITNESSGRAM* report is also available in a non-computerized format. Teachers using the *FITNESSGRAM* system with students having disabilities should consider using the non-computerized report.

The non-computerized format allows you to enter the test name, the student's score, and an appropriate health-referenced standard. When reporting the performance of the disabled student, you may modify the Healthy Fitness Zone as necessary for each individual.

Modification of the Recognition Program

The recognition system used by *FITNESSGRAM* is *You Stay Active!* This recognition system was developed by The Cooper Institute for Aerobics Research and the American Alliance for Health, Physical Education, Recreation and Dance.

You Stay Active! is based primarily on exercise behaviors rather than fitness performance. The program places its highest priority on the development and reinforcement of health-related behaviors, which are obtainable by all students (see chapter 9).

It is intended that all recognition will be available to all children and youth. Criteria for earning recognition may be adapted to meet individual needs of students as necessary. Most of the events in *You Stay Active!* allow for individual selection of specific physical activity and, therefore, are easily modified.

Part

II

ACTIVITYGRAM

Chapter **7** *ACTIVITYGRAM* Administration

A new feature of *FITNESSGRAM*, Revision 6.0, is the inclusion of physical activity assessments. These assessments were added because of the need to reinforce to children the importance of developing lifetime habits of regular physical activity. While fitness is important, it cannot be maintained unless children are physically active.

There are two opportunities to assess physical activity patterns within the *FITNESSGRAM* program: the *FITNESSGRAM* Physical Activity Questionnaire and the *ACTIVITYGRAM* Physical Activity Recall. In order to use the physical activity assessments, you must have the student application installed and allow the students to enter their own information.

ACTIVITYGRAM Physical Activity Recall

A physical activity assessment forms the basis of the *ACTIVITYGRAM* component of the software package. This assessment provides detailed information about the child's activity habits and prescriptive feedback about how active she should be. The *ACTIVITYGRAM* component was designed to be conducted as an "event" similar in focus and structure to the *FITNESSGRAM* assessments. Instructors are encouraged to provide time in the curriculum to utilize this new evaluation tool.

Because of the cognitive demands of recalling physical activity, it may be difficult for young children to get accurate results. For this reason, we recommend that the *ACTIVITYGRAM* program be used primarily for children in grades 5 and higher. However, if used for educational purposes only and if some training or assistance is provided, it still should be possible for younger children (grades 3 and 4) to obtain meaningful results.

Description

The *ACTIVITYGRAM* assessment is a recall of the child's previous day's physical activity based on a validated physical activity instrument known as the Previous Day Physical Activity Recall (PDPAR) (Weston et al. 1997). In the assessment the child is asked to report his activity levels for each 30 min block of time during the day. The format is designed to accommodate both school and non-school days. Each assessment

ACTIVITYGRAM Pyramid

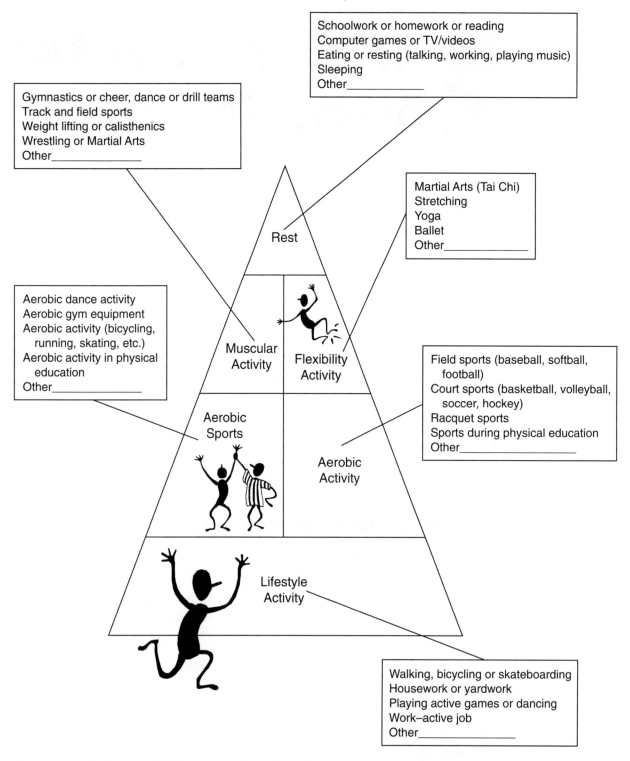

Schoolwork or homework or reading
Computer games or TV/videos
Eating or resting (talking, working, playing music)
Sleeping
Other_____

Gymnastics or cheer, dance or drill teams
Track and field sports
Weight lifting or calisthenics
Wrestling or Martial Arts
Other_____

Martial Arts (Tai Chi)
Stretching
Yoga
Ballet
Other_____

Rest

Aerobic dance activity
Aerobic gym equipment
Aerobic activity (bicycling, running, skating, etc.)
Aerobic activity in physical education
Other_____

Muscular
Activity

Flexibility
Activity

Field sports (baseball, softball, football)
Court sports (basketball, volleyball, soccer, hockey)
Racquet sports
Sports during physical education
Other_____

Aerobic
Sports

Aerobic
Activity

Lifestyle
Activity

Walking, bicycling or skateboarding
Housework or yardwork
Playing active games or dancing
Work–active job
Other_____

Figure 7.1 Options available for physical activity recall.

begins at 7:00 A.M. and continues until 11:00 P.M. For each 30 min time block the child is asked to report the predominant activity for that interval. To help prompt the responses, the children are provided with a list of the common activities. The activities are divided into categories based on the concept of the Activity Pyramid (Lifestyle, Aerobic Activity, Aerobic Sports, Muscular Activity, Flexibility and Rest) (see figure 7.1).

If a student selects an activity from an active category (a category other than Rest), she is prompted to indicate whether she was active in this (or another) activity for "all of the time" or just "some of the time." This distinction improves the accuracy of the assessment and also reinforces to the child that activity does not have to be continuous or done for long periods of time.

For each activity from an active category (a category other than Rest) students are also asked to rate the intensity of the activity (Light, Moderate, Vigorous). The descriptors for the intensity levels were selected to be consistent with current physical activity guidelines that describe recommended levels of moderate and vigorous physical activity. Children may not be familiar with these terms, so make an effort to teach children how to distinguish among these categories. The descriptions in table 7.1 are intended to help children understand these different levels.

Administration

The Physical Activity Recall is accessed through the *ACTIVITYGRAM* module of the student application of the *FITNESSGRAM* software. As previously

mentioned, this module was designed to be administered as an "event" similar to *FITNESSGRAM*. This distinction is important since it sets the tone for how the children and staff at the school will respond to it. By establishing it as an important part of the curriculum, children will put forth a better effort and there will be more cooperation with other teachers regarding scheduling and completing the assessments.

The event would ideally take place during a one- or two-week time span, although it could be administered intermittently or repeatedly during the school year. The key consideration is to provide time for children to complete at least two (preferably three) days of assessment. For the assessment to reflect a child's normal physical activity levels, activity must be assessed on both school days (weekday) and non-school days (weekend or holidays).

Like fitness testing, it is important to follow a standardized protocol and administer the *ACTIVITYGRAM* assessment in a consistent manner across classes and over time. Just as many teachers have students practice the *FITNESSGRAM* tests prior to evaluation, teachers should also help students prepare for the *ACTIVITYGRAM*. Practice assessment sheets that feature a short block of time after school have been included in appendix C to facilitate this training. A recording form is also available (appendix C) to provide a place for children to log their activity levels on the day of their assessment. If this form is used, students will be able to look at their log while completing the assessment. This will greatly facilitate their recall of this day's activity.

Table 7.1 Guidelines for Levels of Physical Activity

Light	Moderate	Vigorous (hard)
Little or no movement, no increase in breathing rate, easy	Movement equal in intensity to a brisk walk, some increase in breathing rate, not too difficult	Moving quickly, breathing hard, hard effort level

Note: Rest is defaulted to an intensity level of Very Light.

Chapter ■8■ Interpreting *ACTIVITYGRAM* Results

The *ACTIVITYGRAM* Physical Activity Recall provides detailed information about the child's normal physical activity patterns. If the children complete at least two days of assessments, the results are printed as the *ACTIVITYGRAM* report. The report includes information regarding the amount of activity performed, activity patterns throughout the day, and the type of activities performed as classified by the Activity Pyramid. (See figure 8.1 for a sample *ACTIVITYGRAM* report). For best results, you should discuss the components of the report with the students during class. Details regarding the interpretation of each of these components is described below.

Minutes of Physical Activity

The most commonly used guidelines for physical activity in children recommend 30 to 60 minutes of moderately intense activity on most days of the week (COPEC guidelines; Pangrazi, Corbin, and Welk 1996). Guidelines for adolescents are similar with respect to moderately intense activity but also advocate participation in some fairly vigorous activity on at least 3 days a week (Sallis and Patrick 1994).

The approach taken in the *ACTIVITYGRAM* report is to focus on the attainment of regular, moderately intense physical activity. The reason for this is that it is a consistent goal for all children (and adults) and also because it is more amenable to the nature of the assessment. The Healthy Activity Zone is set at three bouts of activity (total of 45 min) for children and two bouts of activity (total of 30 min) for adolescents. The reason for including more for elementary students is that they have more discretionary time and are also more likely to get activity through physical education than students in a secondary school. No distinction is made between Moderate and Vigorous activity in this assessment. This reinforces to children that physical activity is for everyone and that activity doesn't have to be vigorous to be beneficial.

Time Profile

The time profile indicates the times when students reported being physically active. Bouts of Moderate and Vigorous activity would correspond to levels 3 and 4 on the

ACTIVITYGRAM

ADAM BODENSTEIN
ACTIVITYGRAM - 4/13/99
Madison County Elementary School

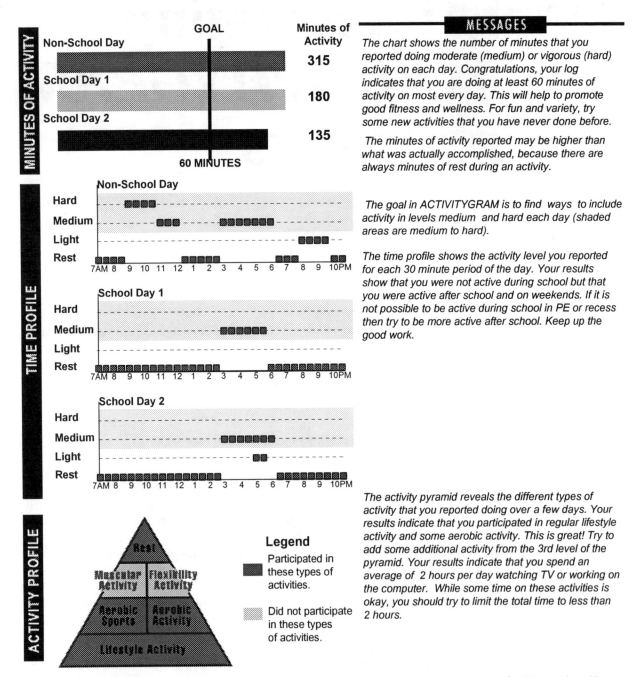

MESSAGES

The chart shows the number of minutes that you reported doing moderate (medium) or vigorous (hard) activity on each day. Congratulations, your log indicates that you are doing at least 60 minutes of activity on most every day. This will help to promote good fitness and wellness. For fun and variety, try some new activities that you have never done before.

The minutes of activity reported may be higher than what was actually accomplished, because there are always minutes of rest during an activity.

The goal in ACTIVITYGRAM is to find ways to include activity in levels medium and hard each day (shaded areas are medium to hard).

The time profile shows the activity level you reported for each 30 minute period of the day. Your results show that you were not active during school but that you were active after school and on weekends. If it is not possible to be active during school in PE or recess then try to be more active after school. Keep up the good work.

The activity pyramid reveals the different types of activity that you reported doing over a few days. Your results indicate that you participated in regular lifestyle activity and some aerobic activity. This is great! Try to add some additional activity from the 3rd level of the pyramid. Your results indicate that you spend an average of 2 hours per day watching TV or working on the computer. While some time on these activities is okay, you should try to limit the total time to less than 2 hours.

ACTIVITYGRAM provides information about your normal levels of physical activity. The report shows what types of activity you do and how often you do them. It includes information that you reported for two or three days during one week.

ACTIVITYGRAM is a module within FITNESSGRAM 6.0 software. FITNESSGRAM materials are distributed by the American Fitness Alliance, a division of Human Kinetics. www.americanfitness.net

©The Cooper Institute for Aerobics Resear

Figure 8.1 Sample *ACTIVITYGRAM* computer report.

graphical report. Emphasis in the interpretation of the time profile should be placed on helping students identify times when they could be more active. Because school time is often out of a student's control, the feedback for this section highlights activity patterns after school and on weekends. For a child to be considered "active" on this section of the report, she must have at least one bout of activity after school and two on the weekends. Feedback can be provided individually or to the class to help them identify times when they could be more active.

Activity Profile

The Activity Profile categorizes the types of activities performed by the child based on the conceptual categories from the Activity Pyramid (Corbin and Pangrazi 1998). Ideally, children would have some activity at each level of the pyramid. Lifestyle activity is recommended for all students (and adults). If students are not performing much activity, it is recommended to first try promoting lifestyle activity. From a health perspective, aerobic activity on the second level can correct for a lack of lifestyle activity on the first level but it is still desirable to promote lifestyle activity among all students. No distinctions are needed between the two types of aerobic activity on the second level. Some children may prefer aerobic activities whereas others may prefer aerobic sports. Participation in either of those categories would ensure that the student is receiving reasonable amounts of aerobic activity. Some distinction can be made at the level of musculoskeletal activity (level 3). Students should perform some activity from each of these categories although there is likely to be some transfer between these categories. Rest is coded at the top of the pyramid because

levels of inactivity should be minimized. The feedback regarding this level does not mention nondiscretionary activities like class, homework, eating, or sleeping. Rather, emphasis is placed on making children (and parents) aware of the child's use of discretionary time. For this reason, feedback is provided for the amount of time spent playing computer games or watching television.

When interpreting the results of the *ACTIVITYGRAM*, it is important to acknowledge the limitations of this assessment. Physical activity assessments are, in general, an inexact science and the *ACTIVITYGRAM* is no exception. In addition to problems with recall, there are additional difficulties that complicate this type of assessment. Children have inherently sporadic activity patterns that are difficult to capture with a self-report instrument. The instrument provides a limited list of possible activities and relies on categorization of activity into discrete time intervals. This may not reflect the normal patterns of children. An additional limitation is that the results of this assessment may not generalize to the child's normal activity pattern. *ACTIVITYGRAM* reflects only 2 to 3 days of activity, and experts agree that it requires about 14 days of monitoring to accurately represent normal activity habits. While these limitations may influence the accuracy of the test, they do not detract from the educational value they contribute in the curriculum.

The recommendation here is to acknowledge the limitations of the instrument and use it for its primary function: teaching children about physical activity. Even if results are not completely accurate, the task of reflecting on their activity habits will provide children with a valuable educational experience.

Part

III

Promoting Physical Activity

Chapter 9 | Recognition and Motivation The *You Stay Active!* Program

An integral part of fitness programs is providing motivation to children and youth, which will encourage them to participate in the activity necessary to produce the desired fitness outcomes. One method of motivating participants is to recognize them for their successes. Recognition can be provided in a variety of ways.

Both theory and practical experience make it obvious that the best way to encourage lifetime health and fitness is to recognize children and youth who establish regular physical activity behavior. The Cooper Institute for Aerobics Research and the American Alliance for Health, Physical Education, Recreation and Dance have developed a recognition program that focuses on active lifestyles designed to produce fitness among children and youth. This program is entitled *You Stay Active!*

You Stay Active! is referred to as a recognition program rather than an awards program because awards often are perceived to be something that is given rather than earned and because awards may be perceived as something only a select few can receive. The goal is to recognize all children and youth who are physically active and who achieve the Healthy Fitness Zone, not to give awards to a few high achievers.

The basis of the recognition is usually fitness performance (the product) or regular activity (the process). Children and youth who are consistently active (do the process) will achieve good fitness (the product) to the extent that heredity, maturation, and other factors allow. You are strongly encouraged to make process recognition the basis of their motivational efforts. Performance recognition is also acceptable but generally should not be used to the exclusion of recognition for being regularly active. High fitness levels on test day are of no value unless the child continues to be active throughout life. The most highly skilled, highly fit students will become unfit adults unless they enjoy activity and continue to be active.

Research indicates that only 10 to 20% of adults participate in adequate levels of regular physical activity (U.S. Department of Health and Human Services 1996). It is obvious that programs used during the last 30 years relying exclusively on the recognition of fitness performance for motivation have not accomplished the goal of encouraging participation in lifelong activity. It is time, perhaps, to consider a change.

You Stay Active! provides numerous tools to use in recognizing students for physical activity. It is primarily a collection of numerous physical activity events that are designed to encourage children and youth to participate in regular physical activity. The system consists of five general types of events which are

- comprehensive activity programs,
- assessment activities,
- cognitive activities,
- other activity promoting events, and
- goal setting performance recognition.

Highlights of the system include:

- Materials for grades K-12
- More than 20 different events
- Handbook includes more than 100 blackline (copy) masters of items such as certificates, activity logs, activity calendars and newsletter

There is also a Model School/Teacher Recognition Program that provides recognition to schools and teachers for conducting programs that focus attention on regular physical activity. Teachers and schools must meet specific criteria to be eligible.

These programs are available by calling The Cooper Institute at 1-800-635-7050.

Funding the Recognition Program

You Stay Active! was designed so that the cost would be minimal. The notebook contains brief descriptive information and more than 100 blackline (copy) masters enabling you to make materials for as many students as you wish without additional expense.

If your budget will not allow the school to purchase a *You Stay Active!* notebook, alternate sources of funding may be available. The following groups may be able to assist in providing recognition items for your students:

- Parent Teacher Association / Parent Teacher Organization
- Community service clubs (Kiwanis, Rotary, Lions, etc.)
- Local businesses

Local businesses and service clubs many times are quite interested in assisting with a school-related project, especially when it will impact students throughout the community. When approaching other organizations, be certain to explain the following concepts of *FITNESSGRAM*, Physical Best, and *You Stay Active!*:

- Health-related approach
- Comparison of students to standards rather than to each other
- Emphasis on development of exercise behavior rather than performance
- High probability for motivating all students with reasonable standards and goals

Rationale

The rationale for the *You Stay Active!* system of recognition is based on the following evidence.

• To be effective, recognition must be based on achievement of goals that are challenging yet attainable (Locke and Lathan 1985). Goals that are too hard are not motivating and can result in lack of effort (Harter 1978). This is especially true for students with low physical self-esteem, often the children and youth who are in most need of improved fitness. Challenging yet achievable goals are intrinsically motivating.

• If a recognition system is not based on goals that seem attainable, children and youth will not be motivated to give effort (Harter 1978). When effort ceases to pay off, children may develop "learned helplessness." Learned helplessness occurs when children perceive that there is no reason to try because trying does not result in reaching the goal. The best way to treat learned helplessness is to reward mastery attempts (effort or process) rather than mastery (performance or product).

• Intrinsic motivation for any behavior, including exercise and physical fitness behaviors, must be based on continuous feedback of progress (information). Awards that are perceived as controlling rather than informative do not build intrinsic motivation (Biddle 1986, Whitehead and Corbin 1991a). Awards based on test performance provide little feedback concerning the person's progress toward the goal. Recognition of behavior can provide day to day feedback in terms of progress and information about personal achievement and competence that can be intrinsically motivating. Intrinsic motivation is evidenced by feelings of competence, willingness to give effort, a perception that exercise is important, lack of anxiety in activity, and enjoyment of activity (Whitehead and Corbin 1991b).

• Awards given to those with exceptionally high scores on fitness tests will often go to those who have the gift of exceptional heredity or early maturity and who are already receiving many rewards for their physical accomplishments (Krahenbuhl et al. 1985, Corbin et al. 1987, Corbin et al. 1990). Research indicates that awards or recognition given for exceptional performance are available to very small numbers of people. The result is a loss of motivation among many.

You Stay Active! focuses on and encourages regular activity. It establishes goals that are possible for all children to attain. Used properly it can make fitness testing and activity an enjoyable experience and a logical extension of daily fitness behavior. It provides the basis for sound education about essential fitness concepts and motivation to become and stay fit for a lifetime.

Chapter 10 The Role of Physical Education

Over the years, the goals and objectives of physical education have evolved to fit the prevailing public health views regarding fitness to health and well-being. Recently, there has been a strong shift in public health policy towards the importance of regular physical activity for optimal health (U.S. Department of Health and Human Services 1996). While physical fitness is still considered an important goal for the public, the general consensus is that it is more important to focus on promoting the process (behavior) of physical activity rather than the product (outcome) of fitness. This shift has brought about a change in the stated goals of physical education. Accordingly, Pate and Hohn (1994) suggest that the mission of physical education is to "... *promote in youngsters the adoption of a physically active lifestyle that persists throughout adulthood"* (italics mine). While physical fitness is still considered a desirable outcome, the emphasis has clearly shifted to a focus on physical activity promotion. A primary reason for this is that physical activity has the potential to track into adulthood (Malina 1996, Pate et al. 1996); fitness, on the other hand, is transient. Students who develop high levels of fitness during their school years will probably not be physically fit at age 50 if they do not continue to participate in regular physical activity. Thus, the key role of physical education is to promote lifetime physical activity.

Communicating the importance of physical activity to children may be difficult if fitness testing is used as the sole form of evaluation in the physical education curriculum. For example, if a child scores well on fitness testing without being active, he may believe that it is not necessary to be active on a regular basis. Conversely, children who are active but score poorly on fitness tests may lose confidence and develop negative attitudes toward physical activity. To promote lifetime physical activity it is important to provide instruction and reinforcement directly on the behavior rather than on the intended outcome. The incorporation of activity messages into the *FITNESSGRAM* module and the development of the behaviorally based *ACTIVITYGRAM* module can help to facilitate this shift in conceptual focus within physical education.

While children can learn about the relationships between physical activity and physical fitness through the interactive *FITNESSGRAM* software, it is incumbent upon the physical education teacher to promote physical activity among the children. Because of limited time constraints, the promotion of physical activity must extend beyond the school and the school day and into the home and community. In this view, the role of physical education broadens to include outreach goals that integrate school, family, and community programs. The purpose of this section is to describe factors that may be important for the promotion of physical activity in children. Emphasis will be placed on how they can be facilitated through physical education.

The Youth Physical Activity Promotion Model

A model of youth activity promotion was recently proposed to explain interactions among different factors thought to influence physical activity in children (Welk 1999). The model distinguishes among factors thought to predispose, enable, and reinforce activity behavior in children (figure 10.1).

Predisposing factors are those things that predispose a child to want to be physically active. This model reduces physical activity behavior into two fundamental questions: "Is it worth it?" and "Am I able?" "Is it worth it?" addresses the benefits vs. costs of participating in physical activity. This question reflects children's attitudes to physical activity

and the level of enjoyment they get from movement experiences. "Am I able?" addresses perceptions of competence. A child can value physical activity but may not want to do it unless she feels capable of performing the activity competently. Children that can answer "yes" to both questions are likely to be predisposed to physical activity.

Enabling factors are those things that enable a child to be physically active. This dimension includes environmental variables such as access to facilities, equipment, and programs that provide opportunities for physical activity. These variables directly influence a child's level of physical activity but do not ensure participation. Children that have access may not choose to make use of their resources, but if children do not have access they do not even have that opportunity. Physical skills and level of physical fitness are also considered enabling factors. Children who are physically fit and skilled are more likely to seek out opportunities to be active while children with poor fitness and skills are less likely to seek out these opportunities. This effect is most likely transmitted through the child's perception of competence ("Am I able?"). A child's perception of competence can have important consequences

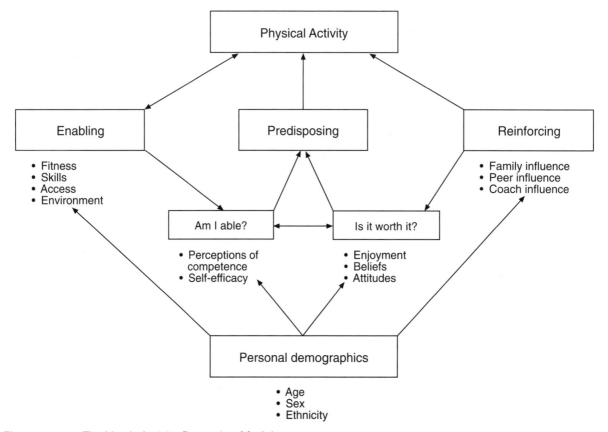

Figure 10.1 The Youth Activity Promotion Model.

Adapted, by permission, from G. Welk, 1999, "The youth physical activity promotion model: a conceptual bridge between theory and practice," *Quest* 51: 5-23.

on a child's attraction to physical activity. Research has even confirmed that perceptions of competence may be more important than actual competence.

Reinforcing factors are the variables that reinforce a child's interest and involvement in physical activity. Parents, peers, teachers, and coaches can all play a role in reinforcing a child's activity behavior. Reinforcing factors can influence a child's physical activity behavior directly and indirectly. The direct effect may stem from active encouragement by a parent or teacher to be physically active. The indirect effect stems from forces that shape a child's predisposition to physical activity. Reinforcement can shape a child's interest in physical activity ("Is it worth it?") as well as his perceptions of competence ("Am I able?"). At young ages, children may be more responsive to influence from teachers and parents. At older ages, peer influence probably exerts a greater influence.

Applying the Youth Physical Activity Promotion Model

The paths proposed in the figure 10.1 suggest that physical activity can be promoted in a variety of ways. The central influence on activity behavior is from the predisposing factors since this domain reflects the child's personal attitudes and perceptions of physical activity. Therefore, emphasis in physical education should be placed on experiences that promote a child's interest and enjoyment in physical activity ("It is worth it!") and perception of competence ("I am able!"). The recent COPEC guidelines (Council for Physical Education for Children 1998) provide valuable suggestions to ensure that physical activities are developmentally appropriate for children. Instructors are encouraged to seek out these and other resources to help create programs that are educationally and motivationally sound for children.

An important point with respect to the physical education curriculum is the need for a hierarchical curriculum that builds with each passing year. The conceptual diagram in figure 10.2 highlights the focus and objectives at each level of development. At a young age, children should be taught a variety of physical skills. With a broader repertoire of physical skills, children will have a greater chance of finding activities that they feel competent in and enjoy. At the middle school level, focus should shift to skill instruction so children can master specific movement skills. Care should be used to minimize experiences of failure since long-term attitudes may begin to form at these ages. In high school, greater emphasis is needed on behavioral skills (self-monitoring, self-reinforcement, and program planning).

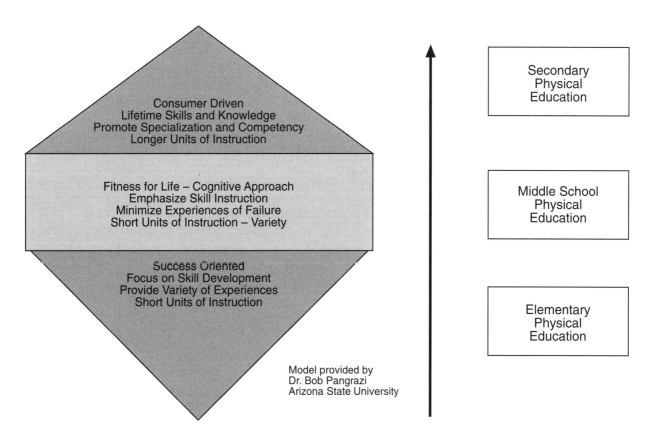

Figure 10.2 A hierarchical model of physical education.

These skills are essential in maintaining lifelong patterns of physical activity. The key concept in this diagram is that the scope of activities and nature of instruction broadens through elementary school and into middle school and then tapers off into high school. Although each teacher may be involved with only a few grade levels, all teachers need to understand the progression of experiences recommended in physical education.

In addition to developing a sound curriculum in school, teachers should consider ways that they can promote physical activity outside of school. Collaborative efforts between schools and community programs are highlighted in the CDC's recently released *Guidelines for School and Community Physical Activity Programs* (Centers for Disease Control and Prevention 1997). Specifically, these guidelines recommend that physical activity be promoted through a coordinated school health program and with links established between the school, family, and community. Physical education teachers can and should play a central role in the development of these links. Descriptions of successful programs that fulfill aspects of these guidelines are described in a new book called *Active Youth* (1998). Resources that can be used to promote physical activity are also available through the *You Stay Active!* program (see chapter 9).

Summary

FITNESSGRAM has been rooted in the philosophy that health (H) is for everyone (E), is for a lifetime (L), and is personal (P). The primary objective of a fitness development program should be to establish regular activity habits through enjoyable fitness experiences. The overall, long-term fitness objective for all students should be to develop or maintain a level of fitness within the Healthy Fitness Zone. Since being healthy is not a meaningful objective for most children, emphasis with children should be on objectives that are more relevant to their daily lives (e.g., looking good and feeling good). At an appropriate age, it is important for all children to understand that physical activity is necessary for good health. A key concept to communicate at this point is that it does not require a tremendous amount of activity or time to maintain a healthy fitness level. Even those students who are not athletes and are not necessarily attracted to physical activity can easily do an adequate amount of activity to be healthy.

The use of *FITNESSGRAM* and *ACTIVITYGRAM* in the curriculum can help communicate these messages about physical activity and health. Some additional recommendations for promoting physical activity and physical fitness within physical education are included below:

• Provide a rationale for children to participate in regular physical activity. Make certain that the reasons are relevant to their daily life. The benefits of looking good, feeling good, and enjoying life more are usually most salient with children.

• Provide feedback regarding current status. Test results should be used for education on physical activity and fitness and to select areas for improving or maintaining good performance.

• Encourage students to establish short-term and long-term goals. Short-term goals are probably the most important and should be goals related to physical activity rather than goals related to fitness achievement. Instead of a goal to do 5 more sit-ups on the next test, a more appropriate process goal would be to perform abdominal strengthening activities 3-4 times each week. If a student works hard toward improving his fitness but does not manage to achieve the "product" goal, the result is a feeling of failure. A process goal would allow the student to achieve success while slowly making progress toward the desired result. Goal-setting forms are included in appendix C.

• Help each student identify a regular time and place to fit physical activity into the daily schedule. Talk about fitting activities into daily routines such as walking or biking to school, to a friend's house, or to the store. Part of making time for activity may be less time watching TV or playing video games.

• Have students make a written commitment to participate in the activity required to achieve the goal. The activity should be enjoyable to the student. The list of activities should be a specific listing of type of activity, day of the week, time of day, place, and other specific details.

• Encourage students to keep track of their participation on some type of exercise log or through the *ACTIVITYGRAM* software.

• Periodically ask students about their progress, showing that you are seriously interested in the program.

• Discuss progress and problems. Being active is not easy. If a student is having difficulty meeting a goal, ask other students to suggest solutions.

• Praise students for even small accomplishments in their efforts to achieve their goals. Feedback on success is very important in making children feel competent and thus establishing intrinsic motivation.

• Recognize student achievement of activity goals through the use of rewards, awards, stickers on a wall chart, posting names on success charts, etc. (see chapter 9).

• Recommend activities that are of low to moderate intensity since these activities are more likely to be maintained than some team sport activities. Activities such as walking and recreational bike riding are examples.

• Involve parents as much as possible. Teach parents about the important role they play in shaping a child's interest in and enjoyment of physical activity.

• Ideally, families should try to do activities together. Evening and weekend outings are fun and enjoyable. If the whole family cannot participate together, encourage activity in pairs.

• If families do not do activities together, encourage family support. Praise and encouragement are more effective than nagging. Parents can transport children to activity sessions; children can help parents with chores so parents have time for activity.

• Be a role model to your class by including regular activity as a part of your lifestyle. Tell your students about your enjoyment of physical activity and its benefits.

References

American Alliance for Health, Physical Education, Recreation and Dance. 1996. *Physical Best and Children with Disabilities*. Reston, VA: American Alliance for Health, Physical Education, Recreation and Dance.

Biddle, S.J.W. 1986. Exercise motivation: theory and practice. *British Journal of Physical Education* 17: 40-44.

Blair, S.N., Kohl, H.W., Gordon, N.F., and Paffenbarger, R.S. 1992. How much physical activity is good for health? *Annals and Reviews in Public Health* 13: 99-126.

Blair, S.N., Kohl, H.W., Paffenbarger, R.S., Clark, D.G., Cooper, K.H., and Gibbons, L.W. 1989. Physical fitness and all-cause mortality. *Journal of the American Medical Association* 262: 2395-2437.

Blair, S.N., Clark, D.G., Cureton, K.J., and Powell, K.E. 1989. Exercise and fitness in childhood: Implications for a lifetime of health. In *Perspectives in Exercise Science and Sports Medicine: Volume 2 Youth Exercise and Sports*, C.V. Gisolfi & Lamb, D.R. eds. pp. 401-430 Indianapolis, IN: Benchmark.

Casperson, C.J., Christenson, G.M., and Pollard, R.A. 1986. Status of 1990 physical fitness and exercise objectives - evidence from NHIS 1985. *Public Health Report* 101: 587-592.

Centers for Disease Control and Prevention. 1997. Guidelines for school and community programs to promote lifelong physical activity among young people. *Morbidity and Mortality Weekly Report* 46(RR-6): 1-36.

Council for Physical Education for Children. 1998. *Physical Activity for Children: A Statement of Guidelines*. Reston, VA: NASPE Publications.

Corbin, C.B. 1987. Youth fitness, exercise and health: There is much to be done. *Research Quarterly for Exercise and Sport* 58: 308-314.

Corbin, C.B., Lovejoy, P., Steingard, P., and Emerson, R. 1990. Fitness awards: Do they accomplish their intended objectives? *American Journal of Health Promotion* 4: 345-351.

Corbin, C.B. and Pangrazi, R.P. 1998. Physical activity pyramid rebuffs peak experience. *ACSM's Health and Fitness Journal* 2(1): 12-17.

Epstein, L.H., Valoski, A., Wing, R.R., and McCurly, J. 1990. Ten-year follow-up of behavioral family-based treatment for obese children. *Journal of American Medical Association* 264: 2519-2524.

Gortmaker, S.L., Dietz, W.H., Sobol, A.H. and Wehler, C.A. 1987. Increasing pediatric obesity in the U.S. *American Journal of Diseases of Children* 1: 535-540.

Harter, S. 1978. Effectance motivation revisited. *Child Development* 21: 34-64.

Human Kinetics. 1998. *Active Youth: Ideas for Implementing CDC Physical Activity Promotion Guidelines*, Champaign, IL: Human Kinetics.

Johnston, F.W., Hamill, D.V. and Lemeshow, S. 1974. *Skinfold Thickness of Children 12-17 Years, Series 11, No. 132*. Washington, D.C.: U.S. Center for Health Statistics.

Johnston, F.W., Hamill, D.V. and Lemeshow, S. 1972. *Skinfold Thickness of Children 6-11 Years, Series 11, No. 120*. Washington, D.C.: U.S. Center for Health Statistics.

Kline, G.M., Porcari, J.P., Hintermeister, R., Freedson, P.S., Ward, A., McCarron, R.F., Ross, J. and Rippe, J.M. 1987. Estimation of VO_2max from a one-mile track walk, gender, age, and body weight. *Medicine and Science in Sports and Exercise* 19 (3): 253-259.

Krahenbuhl, G.S., Skinner, J.S., and Kohrt, W.M. 1985. Developmental aspects of maximal aerobic power in children. *Exercise Sport Science Review* 13: 503-538.

Leger, L.A., Mercier, D., Gadoury, C. and Lambert, J. 1988. The multistage 20 metre shuttle run test for aerobic fitness. *Journal of Sport Sciences* 6: 93-101.

Leger, L. and Lambert, J. 1982. A maximal 20-m shuttle run test to predict VO_2max. *European Journal of Applied Physiology* 49: 1-12.

Locke, E.A. and Lathan, G.P. 1985. The application of goal setting to sports. *Journal of Sport Psychology* 7: 205-222.

Lohman, T.G. 1987. The use of skinfold to estimate body fatness in children and youth. *Journal of Physical Education, Recreation and Dance* 58: 98-102.

Lohman, T.G. 1992. *Advances in body composition*. Champaign, IL: Human Kinetics Publishers.

Malina, R.M. 1996. Tracking of physical activity and physical fitness across the lifespan. *Research Quarterly for Exercise and Sport* 67(3): 48-57.

Massicote, D. 1990. *Project # 240-0010-88/89: Partial Curl-up, push-ups, and multistage 20 meter shuttle run, national norms for 6 to 17 year-olds*. Montreal, Canada: Canadian Association for Health, Physical Education and Recreation and Fitness and Amateur Sport Canada.

McSwegin, P.J., Plowman, S.A., Wolff, G.M. and Guttenberg, G.L. 1998. The validity of a one-mile walk test for high school age individuals. *Measurement in Physical Education and Exercise Science* 2 (1): 47-63.

Pangrazi, R.P., Corbin, C.B. and Welk, G.J. 1996. Physical activity for children and youth. *Journal of Physical Education, Recreation and Dance* 67 (4):38-43.

Pate, R.R., Baranowski, T., Dowda, M., and Trost, S.G. 1996. Tracking of physical activity in young children. *Medicine and Science in Sports and Exercise* 28(1): 92-96.

Pate, R.R., and Hohn, R.C. 1994. A contemporary mission for physical education. In *Health and fitness through physical education*, edited by R. R. Pate and R. C. Hohn. Champaign, IL: Human Kinetics.

Pate, R.R., Ross, J.G., Dotson, C. and Gilbert, G.G. 1985. The new norms: A comparison with the 1980 AAHPERD norms. *Journal of Physical Education, Recreation and Dance* 56: 28-30.

Ross, J.G., Pate, R.R., Lohman, T.G., and Christenson, G.M. 1987. Changes in the body composition of children. *Journal of Physical Education, Recreation and Dance* 58: 74-77.

Sallis, J.F. and Patrick, K. 1994. Physical activity guidelines for adolescents: consensus statement. *Pediatric Exercise Science* 6: 302-314.

Schiemer, Sue. 1996. The pacer - a really fun run. In *Ideas for Action II: More Award Winning Approaches to Physical Activity*. Reston, VA: American Alliance for Health, Physical Education, Recreation and Dance.

Slaughter, M.H., Lohman, T.G., Boileau, R.A., Horswill, C.A., Stillman, R.J., Van Loan, M.D. and Benben, D.A. 1988. Skinfold equations for estimation of body fatness in children and youth. *Human Biology* 60: 709-723.

Troiano, R.P., Flegal, K.M., Kuczmarski, Campbell, S.M. and Johnson, C.L. 1995. Overweight prevalence and trends for children and adolescents. *Archives of Pediatric and Adolescent Medicine* 149: 1085-1091.

Troiano, R.P., and Flegal, K.M. 1998. Overweight children and adolescents: Description, epidemiology, and demographics. *Pediatrics* 101 (3): 497-504.

U.S. Department of Health and Human Services.1996. *Physical Activity and Health: A Report of the Surgeon General*. Atlanta, GA: U.S. Department of Health and Human Services, Centers for Disease Control and Prevention, & National Center for Chronic Disease Prevention and Health Promotion.

Welk, G.J. 1999. The youth physical activity promotion model: A conceptual bridge between theory and practice. *Quest* 51: 5-23.

Weston, A.T., Petosa, R. and Pate, R.R. 1997. Validation of an instrument for measurement of physical activity in youth. *Medicine and Science in Sports and Exercise* 29 (1): 138-143.

Whitehead, J.R. and Corbin, C.B. 1991a. Effects of fitness test type, teacher, and gender on exercise intrinsic motivation and physical self-worth. *Journal of School Health* 61: 11-16.

Whitehead, J.R. and Corbin, C.B. 1991b. Youth fitness testing: The effects of percentile-based evaluative feedback on intrinsic motivation. *Research Quarterly for Exercise and Sport* 62: 225-231.

Willaims, D.P., Going, S.B., Lohman, T.G., Harsha, D.W., Webber, L.S., and Bereson, G.S. 1992. Body fatness and the risk of elevated blood pressure, total cholesterol and serum lipoprotein ratios in children and youth. *American Journal of Public Health* 82: 358-363.

Winnick, J.P. and Short, F.X. 1985. *Physical fitness testing of the disabled: Project unique*. Champaign, IL: Human Kinetics Publishers.

Appendix A
Information on Testing Equipment

Sources of Testing Equipment

The PACER Music CD or audiocassette

American Fitness Alliance
P.O. Box 5076
Champaign, IL 61825-5076
1-800-747-4457

Skinfold Calipers

Lange Skinfold Calipers
Country Technology
P.O. Box 87
Gay Mills, WI 54631
608-735-4718
Adipometers
American Fitness Alliance
P.O. Box 5076
Champaign, IL 61825-5076
1-800-747-4457

Fat Control, Inc.
P.O. Box 10117
Towson, MD 21204
717-993-3550

Training Films on Skinfold Measurement

American Fitness Alliance
P.O. Box 5076
Champaign, IL 61825-5076
1-800-747-4457

Curl-Up Measuring Strips

American Fitness Alliance
P.O. Box 5076
Champaign, IL 61825-5076
1-800-747-4457

Measuring Strip for Curl-Up Test

Cut from poster board.

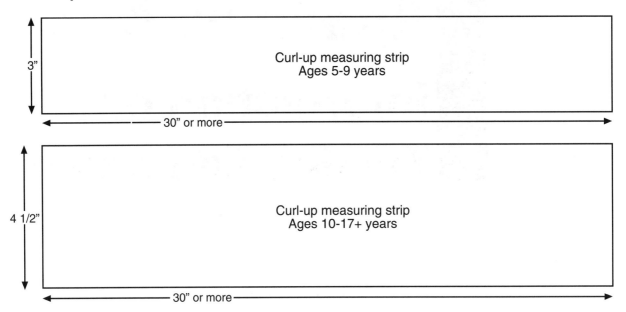

Other Suggestions for Measuring Curl-Up Distances

There are any number of methods to measure the distance traveled in the curl-up test. The important factor is to ensure that the student is moving the fingertips 3″ for ages 5-9 years and $4\frac{1}{2}$″ for ages 10-17+. Another factor to consider is that the student should be able to "feel" the stopping point rather than rely on "seeing" it. Do not be afraid to experiment with other methods to measure this distance.

1. Use tape and a pencil to indicate the marks. Put tape on the mat at the starting point for the fingertips. Tape a pencil to the mat parallel to the starting line at the stopping point (3″ or $4\frac{1}{2}$″).

2. Use tape and a yardstick to indicate the marks. Put tape on the mat at the starting point for the fingertips. Have the third partner standing astride the person doing curl-ups secure a yardstick placed on the mat under the knees and parallel to the starting line. The yardstick should be placed either 3″ or $4\frac{1}{2}$″ from the starting line.

3. Permanent measuring strips like those pictured above could be cut from a sheet of $\frac{1}{4}$″ plywood. These would need to be carefully sanded to prevent splinters. Laminated poster board would also provide more permanent measuring strips.

4. Measuring cards could be cut to the appropriate width (3″ or $4\frac{1}{2}$″) out of index cards. Two would be needed for every two students. Cards would need to be taped to the mat in position for the student to slide the fingers from one edge of the card to the other.

Equipment for Modified Pull-Up

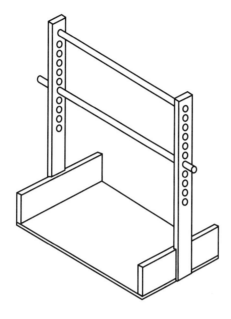 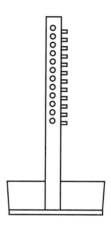

Items needed:

Two 2 × 4 × 48 in. pieces for uprights

Two 2 × 8 × 24 in. pieces for base of uprights

One ³/₄ in. plywood 24 × 39 in. for support platform

One 1¹/₈ in. steel pipe for chinning bar at least 43" long

One 1 ¹/₄ in. dowel for top support 39" long

Twenty-four ³/₈ in. dowel pieces cut 3¹/₂ in. long Nails, wood screws, and wood glue for construction.

1. Beginning 2¹/₂ in. from the top end of each 2 × 4 × 48 piece, drill one hole through the 2 in. thickness for the 1¹/₄ in. dowel support rod.

2. Drill eleven more 1 ¹/₈ in. holes below the first hole, spaced 2 ¹/₂ in. from center to center, in each piece for the steel pipe.

3. Beginning 3³/₄ in. from the top of these upright pieces, drill twelve ³/₈ in. holes into the 4 in. thickness for the dowel pieces. Center these holes between the holes for the steel pipe.

4. Assemble the pieces and finish with polyurethane or shellac.

Equipment for Back-Saver Sit and Reach

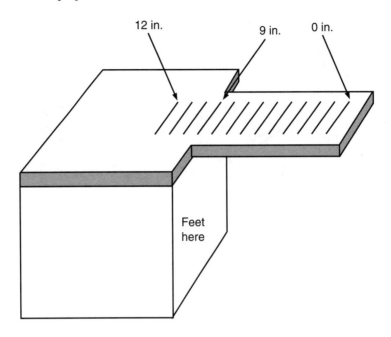

1. Using any sturdy wood or comparable material (³/₄ in. plywood seems to work well) cut the following pieces:

Two pieces 12 × 12 in.

Two pieces 12 × 10¹/₂ in.

One piece 12 × 22 in.

2. Cut 10 × 4 in. pieces from each side of one end of the 12 × 22 in. piece to make the top of the box. Beginning at the small end, mark 1 in. intervals up to 12 in.

3. Construct a box (use nails, screws, or wood glue) with the remaining four pieces. Attach the top. It is crucial that the 9 in. mark be exactly parallel with the vertical plane against which the subject's foot will be placed. The 0 in. marks the end nearest the subject.

4. Cover the apparatus with polyurethane sealer or shellac.

Alternate Flexibility Testing Apparatus

1. Use a sturdy cardboard box at least 12 in. tall. Turn the box so that the bottom is up. Tape a yardstick to the bottom. The yardstick must be placed so that the 9 in. mark is exactly parallel with the vertical plane against which the subject's foot will be placed and the 0 in. end is nearer the subject.

2. Use a bench that is about 12 in. wide. Turn the bench on its side. Tape a yardstick to the bench so that the 9 in. mark is exactly parallel with the vertical plane against which the subject's foot will be placed and the 0 in. end is nearer the subject.

Appendix B
Physical Activity Guidelines

Physical Activity Guidelines for Children and Adolescents

Children's Physical Activity Guidelines
(based on COPEC 1998)

- Guideline 1: Elementary school-aged children should accumulate at least 30-60 minutes of age and developmentally appropriate physical activity on most days of the week.

- Guideline 2: An accumulation of more than 60 minutes is encouraged for children.

- Guideline 3: Some of the child's activity each day should include moderate to vigorous activity in periods lasting 10-15 minutes.

- Guideline 4: Extended periods of inactivity are inappropriate for children.

- Guideline 5: A variety of activities from the Physical Activity Pyramid are recommended for children.

Adolescent's Physical Activity Guidelines
(based on Sallis, Patrick, and Long 1994)

- Guideline 1: All adolescents should be physically active daily, or nearly every day, as part of play, games, sports, work, transportation, recreation, physical education, or planned exercise, in the context of family, school, and community activities.

- Guideline 2: Adolescents should engage in three or more sessions per week of activities that last 20 min or more at a time and that require moderate to vigorous levels of exertion.

Appendix C
Copy Masters

Student Name: _____

Get Fit Conditioning Program

The Get Fit Conditioning Program is a six-week program designed to help you get in shape for your fitness test.

    Guidelines are as follows:

        Participate at least three times each week for six weeks.

        Complete the exercise log and return it to your teacher.

        You may do some of your workouts during your physical education class.

        Select activities from this appendix or do your favorite activities from physical education class.

        Place a check mark in the box for each day you work out. Your workout should include: warm-up, strength development, aerobic activities, and cool-down.

Warm-up— At the beginning of the workout do at least three warm-up exercises. Move easily at first and gradually get faster. Hold a stretch for 10 counts and do not bounce. Be sure to do work for the upper body and the legs.

Strength dev elopment— Do at least three strength exercises. Do as many of each exercise as you can up to 20.

Aerobic activity— Begin with 2 to 5 minutes of your activity and gradually increase the time to 25-30 minutes.

Cool-down— Do three of your favorite activities from this list. Be sure to stretch upper and lower body and trunk.

	Sunday	Monday	Tuesday	Wednesday	Thursday	Friday	Saturday
Week 1 Date:							
Week 2 Date:							
Week 3 Date:							
Week 4 Date:							
Week 5 Date:							
Week 6 Date:							

Source: FITNESSGRAM Test Administration Manual, Second Edition

FITNESSGRAM

FITNESSGRAM Get Fit Exercises

Warm-up Activities

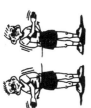

Side Bend

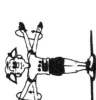
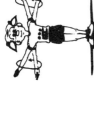

Trunk Twist

Knee Lift

Calf Stretch

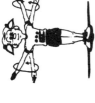

Arm Circles

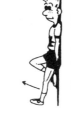
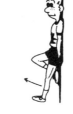
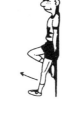
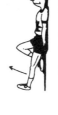

Jumping Jacks

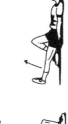

Brisk Walking

Strength Development Activities

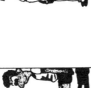

Crunch

Curl-ups

Military Press

Arm Curls

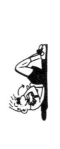

Sit-ups

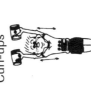

Back Arch

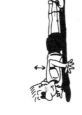
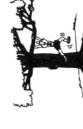
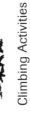

Lunges

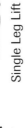

Single Leg Lift

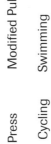

Wall Sit

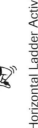

Push-ups

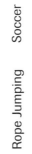

Modified Pull-ups

Horizontal Ladder Activites

Climbing Activities

Aerobic Activities

Jogging Cycling Swimming Brisk Walking Rope Jumping Soccer Basketball

Cool-down Activities

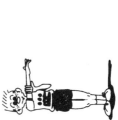
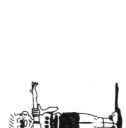
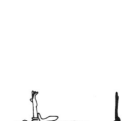

Calf Stretch

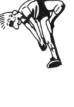

Thigh Stretch

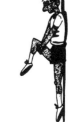

Sitting Toe Touch

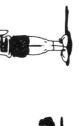

Knee Hug

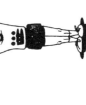

Arm/Shoulder Stretch

Arm/Side Stretch

Source: FITNESSGRAM Test Administration Manual, Second Edition

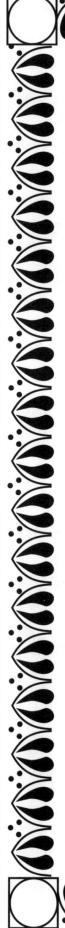

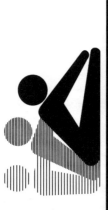

FITNESSGRAM®

GET FIT AWARD

This certifies that

_____

has succesfully completed the "Get Fit" activity program and demonstrated outstanding commitment to developing good fitness habits.

Date _____

Source: FITNESSGRAM Test Administration Manual, Second Edition

Physical Activity Goals

Week of: _____

My plans are to do

	Activity I plan to do	Time of day	Friend(s) who will be active with me
Monday			
Tuesday			
Wednesday			
Thursday			
Friday			
Saturday			
Sunday			

Date _____ **Student's signature** _____ **Teacher's initials** _____

The actual activity I did

	Yes, I did the following activity	How long?	I was unable to do planned activity because
Monday			
Tuesday			
Wednesday			
Thursday			
Friday			
Saturday			
Sunday			

Source: FITNESSGRAM Test Administration Manual, Second Edition

FITNESS CONTRACT

I, _____, agree to:

When I complete the requirements listed above,
I will receive appropriate recognition of my activity.

Student's Signature _____

Date _____

I agree that the student named above will be
recognized for completing the terms of
this contract by receiving

_____

Teacher's Signature _____

Date _____

Source: FITNESSGRAM Test Administration Manual, Second Edition

FITNESSGRAM

The PACER Individual Score Sheet

Teacher _____   Class Period _____   Date _____

Laps (20-meter lengths)

1	1	2	3	4	5	6	7					
2	8	9	10	11	12	13	14	15				
3	16	17	18	19	20	21	22	23				
4	24	25	26	27	28	29	30	31	32			
5	33	34	35	36	37	38	39	40	41			
6	42	43	44	45	46	47	48	49	50	51		
7	52	53	54	55	56	57	58	59	60	61		
8	62	63	64	65	66	67	68	69	70	71	72	
9	73	74	75	76	77	78	79	80	81	82	83	
10	84	85	86	87	88	89	90	91	92	93	94	
11	95	96	97	98	99	100	101	102	103	104	105	106
12	107	108	109	110	111	112	113	114	115	116	117	118
13	119	120	121	122	123	124	125	126	127	128	129	130	131
14	132	133	134	135	136	137	138	139	140	141	142	143	144
15	145	146	147	148	149	150	151	152	153	154	155	156	157

Lane _____   Student Name _____   Laps Completed _____

Source: FITNESSGRAM Test Administration Manual, Second Edition

FITNESSGRAM

The PACER Group Score Sheet

Teacher _____ Class Period _____ Date _____

Laps (20-meter lengths)

1	1	2	3	4	5	6	7						
2	8	9	10	11	12	13	14	15					
3	16	17	18	19	20	21	22	23					
4	24	25	26	27	28	29	30	31	32				
5	33	34	35	36	37	38	39	40	41				
6	42	43	44	45	46	47	48	49	50	51			
7	52	53	54	55	56	57	58	59	60	61			
8	62	63	64	65	66	67	68	69	70	71	72		
9	73	74	75	76	77	78	79	80	81	82	83		
10	84	85	86	87	88	89	90	91	92	93	94		
11	95	96	97	98	99	100	101	102	103	104	105	106	
12	107	108	109	110	111	112	113	114	115	116	117	118	
13	119	120	121	122	123	124	125	126	127	128	129	130	131
14	132	133	134	135	136	137	138	139	140	141	142	143	144
15	145	146	147	148	149	150	151	152	153	154	155	156	157

Lane	Student name	Laps completed	Lane	Student name	Laps completed

Source: FITNESSGRAM Test Administration Manual, Second Edition

One-Mile Run Individual Score Sheet

Runner Name: _____

Scorer Name: _____

Laps Completed (cross off each lap number as your runner completes it)

1	2	3	4	5	6	7	8	9	10
11	12	13	14	15	16	17	18	19	20

Finish Time: _____

Source: FITNESSGRAM Test Administration Manual, Second Edition

✂ —

One-Mile Run Individual Score Sheet

Runner Name: _____

Scorer Name: _____

Laps Completed (cross off each lap number as your runner completes it)

1	2	3	4	5	6	7	8	9	10
11	12	13	14	15	16	17	18	19	20

Finish Time: _____

Source: FITNESSGRAM Test Administration Manual, Second Edition

Walk Test Individual Score Sheet

Runner Name: _____

Scorer Name: _____

Laps Completed (cross off each lap number as your runner completes it)

1	2	3	4	5	6	7	8	9	10
11	12	13	14	15	16	17	18	19	20

Finish Time: _____

Heart Rate: _____

Source: FITNESSGRAM Test Administration Manual, Second Edition

✂ -

Walk Test Individual Score Sheet

Runner Name: _____

Scorer Name: _____

Laps Completed (cross off each lap number as your runner completes it)

1	2	3	4	5	6	7	8	9	10
11	12	13	14	15	16	17	18	19	20

Finish Time: _____

Heart Rate: _____

Source: FITNESSGRAM Test Administration Manual, Second Edition

FITNESSGRAM PACER Test - Individual Score Sheet

Student Name _____ Class _____ Date _____

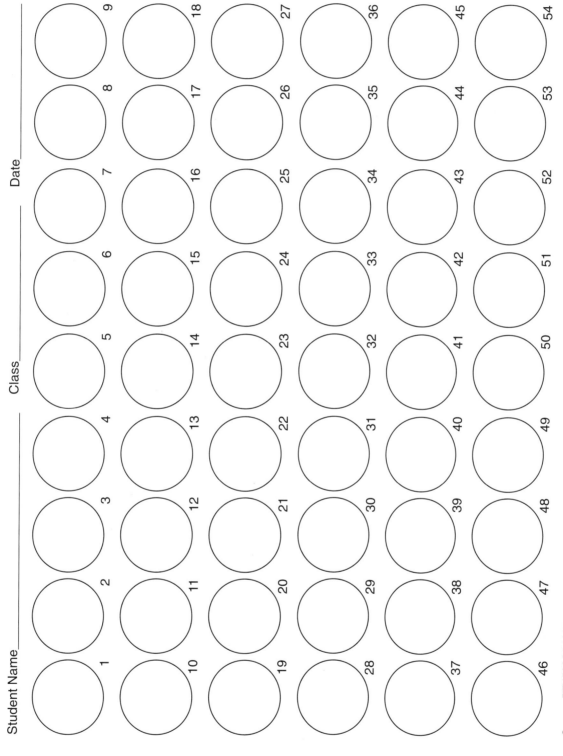

FITNESSGRAM

Body Composition Conversion Chart

BOYS

Total MM	% Fat	Total MM	% Fat	Total MM	% Fat	Total MM	% Fat	Total MM	% Fat
1.0	1.7	16.0	12.8	31.0	23.8	46.0	34.8	61.0	45.8
1.5	2.1	16.5	13.1	31.5	24.2	46.5	35.2	61.5	46.2
2.0	2.5	17.0	13.5	32.0	24.5	47.0	35.5	62.0	46.6
2.5	2.8	17.5	13.9	32.5	24.9	47.5	35.9	62.5	46.9
3.0	3.2	18.0	14.2	33.0	25.3	48.0	36.3	63.0	47.3
3.5	3.6	18.5	14.6	33.5	25.6	48.5	36.6	63.5	47.7
4.0	3.9	19.0	15.0	34.0	26.0	49.0	37.0	64.0	48.0
4.5	4.3	19.5	15.3	34.5	26.4	49.5	37.4	64.5	48.4
5.0	4.7	20.0	15.7	35.0	26.7	50.0	37.8	65.0	48.8
5.5	5.0	20.5	16.1	35.5	27.1	50.5	38.1	65.5	49.1
6.0	5.4	21.0	16.4	36.0	27.5	51.0	38.5	66.0	49.5
6.5	5.8	21.5	16.8	36.5	27.8	51.5	38.9	66.5	49.9
7.0	6.1	22.0	17.2	37.0	28.2	52.0	39.2	67.0	50.2
7.5	6.5	22.5	17.5	37.5	28.6	52.5	39.6	67.5	50.6
8.0	6.9	23.0	17.9	38.0	28.9	53.0	40.0	68.0	51.0
8.5	7.2	23.5	18.3	38.5	29.3	53.5	40.3	68.5	51.3
9.0	7.6	24.0	18.6	39.0	29.7	54.0	40.7	69.0	51.7
9.5	8.0	24.5	19.0	39.5	30.0	54.5	41.1	69.5	52.1
10.0	8.4	25.0	19.4	40.0	30.4	55.0	41.4	70.0	52.5
10.5	8.7	25.5	19.7	40.5	30.8	55.5	41.8	70.5	52.8
11.0	9.1	26.0	20.1	41.0	31.1	56.0	42.2	71.0	53.2
11.5	9.5	26.5	20.5	41.5	31.5	56.5	42.5	71.5	53.6
12.0	9.8	27.0	20.8	42.0	31.9	57.0	42.9	72.0	53.9
12.5	10.2	27.5	21.2	42.5	32.2	57.5	43.3	72.5	54.3
13.0	10.6	28.0	21.6	43.0	32.6	58.0	43.6	73.0	54.7
13.5	10.9	28.5	21.9	43.5	33.0	58.5	44.0	73.5	55.0
14.0	11.3	29.0	22.3	44.0	33.3	59.0	44.4	74.0	55.4
14.5	11.7	29.5	22.7	44.5	33.7	59.5	44.7	74.5	55.8
15.0	12.0	30.0	23.1	45.0	34.1	60.0	45.1	75.0	56.1
15.5	12.4	30.5	23.4	45.5	34.4	60.5	45.5	75.5	56.5

Source: FITNESSGRAM Test Administration Manual, Second Edition

FITNESSGRAM

Body Composition Conversion Chart

GIRLS

Total MM	% Fat	Total MM	% Fat	Total MM	% Fat	Total MM	% Fat	Total MM	% Fat
1.0	5.7	16.0	14.9	31.0	24.0	46.0	33.2	61.0	42.3
1.5	6.0	16.5	15.2	31.5	24.3	46.5	33.5	61.5	42.6
2.0	6.3	17.0	15.5	32.0	24.6	47.0	33.8	62.0	42.9
2.5	6.6	17.5	15.8	32.5	24.9	47.5	34.1	62.5	43.2
3.0	6.9	18.0	16.1	33.0	25.2	48.0	34.4	63.0	43.5
3.5	7.2	18.5	16.4	33.5	25.5	48.5	34.7	63.5	43.8
4.0	7.5	19.0	16.7	34.0	25.8	49.0	35.0	64.0	44.1
4.5	7.8	19.5	17.0	34.5	26.1	49.5	35.3	64.5	44.4
5.0	8.2	20.0	17.3	35.0	26.5	50.0	35.6	65.0	44.8
5.5	8.5	20.5	17.6	35.5	26.8	50.5	35.9	65.5	45.1
6.0	8.8	21.0	17.9	36.0	27.1	51.0	36.2	66.0	45.4
6.5	9.1	21.5	18.2	36.5	27.4	51.5	36.5	66.5	45.7
7.0	9.4	22.0	18.5	37.0	27.7	52.0	36.8	67.0	46.0
7.5	9.7	22.5	18.8	37.5	28.0	52.5	37.1	67.5	46.3
8.0	10.0	23.0	19.1	38.0	28.3	53.0	37.4	68.0	46.6
8.5	10.3	23.5	19.4	38.5	28.6	53.5	37.7	68.5	46.9
9.0	10.6	24.0	19.7	39.0	28.9	54.0	38.0	69.0	47.2
9.5	10.9	24.5	20.0	39.5	29.2	54.5	38.3	69.5	47.5
10.0	11.2	25.0	20.4	40.0	29.5	55.0	38.7	70.0	47.8
10.5	11.5	25.5	20.7	40.5	29.8	55.5	39.0	70.5	48.1
11.0	11.8	26.0	21.0	41.0	30.1	56.0	39.3	71.0	48.4
11.5	12.1	26.5	21.3	41.5	30.4	56.5	39.6	71.5	48.7
12.0	12.4	27.0	21.6	42.0	30.7	57.0	39.9	72.0	49.0
12.5	12.7	27.5	21.9	42.5	31.0	57.5	40.2	72.5	49.3
13.0	13.0	28.0	22.2	43.0	31.3	58.0	40.5	73.0	49.6
13.5	13.3	28.5	22.5	43.5	31.6	58.5	40.8	73.5	49.9
14.0	13.6	29.0	22.8	44.0	31.9	59.0	41.1	74.0	50.2
14.5	13.9	29.5	23.1	44.5	32.2	59.5	41.4	74.5	50.5
15.0	14.3	30.0	23.4	45.0	32.6	60.0	41.7	75.0	50.9
15.5	14.6	30.5	23.7	45.5	32.9	60.5	42.0	75.5	51.2

Source: FITNESSGRAM Test Administration Manual, Second Edition

FITNESSGRAM

Class Score Sheet

Teacher _____

Class _____

Page Number _____ Grade _____

Test Date _____

ID#	Name	Birth date	Sex	Height	Weight	Aerobic capacity	Curl-up	Upper body	Trunk lift	Flexibility		Skinfolds	
										L/R		Triceps	Calf

Source: FITNESSGRAM Test Administration Manual, Second Edition

FITNESSGRAM

Personal Fitness Record

Name _____   Age _____   Height _____   Weight _____   School _____   Grade _____

	Date:		Date:	
	Score	HFZ	Score	HFZ
Aerobic capacity:				
_____				
Curl-up				
Trunk lift				
Upper body strength:				
_____				
Flexibility:				
_____				
Skinfolds:				
Triceps				
Calf				
Total				

Note: HFZ indicates you have performed in the Healthy Fitness Zone.

I understand that my fitness record is personal. I do not have to share my results. My fitness record is important since it allows me to check my fitness level. If it is low, I will need to do more activity. If it is acceptable, I need to continue my current activity level. I know that I can ask my teacher for ideas for improving my fitness level.

Source: FITNESSGRAM Test Administration Manual, Second Edition

FITNESSGRAM

Personal Fitness Record

Name _____   Age _____   Height _____   Weight _____   School _____   Grade _____

	Date:		Date:	
	Score	HFZ	Score	HFZ
Aerobic capacity:				
_____				
Curl-up				
Trunk lift				
Upper body strength:				
_____				
Flexibility:				
_____				
Skinfolds:				
Triceps				
Calf				
Total				

Note: HFZ indicates you have performed in the Healthy Fitness Zone

I understand that my fitness record is personal. I do not have to share my results. My fitness record is important since it allows me to check my fitness level. If it is low, I will need to do more activity. If it is acceptable, I need to continue my current activity level. I know that I can ask my teacher for ideas for improving my fitness level.

Source: FITNESSGRAM Test Administration Manual, Second Edition

FITNESSGRAM

Personal Fitness Record

Name _____ School _____ Age ____ Grade ____ Ht ____ Wt ____

	Date:		Date:		Date:	
	Score	HFZ	Score	HFZ	Score	HFZ
Aerobic capacity:						
_____						
Curl-up						
Trunk lift						
Upper body strength:						
_____						
Flexibility:						
_____						
Skinfolds:						
Triceps						
Calf						
Total						

Note: HFZ indicates you have performed in the Healthy Fitness Zone.

I understand that my fitness record is personal. I do not have to share my results. My fitness record is important since it allows me to check my fitness level. If it is low, I will need to do more activity. If it is acceptable, I need to continue my current activity level. I know that I can ask my teacher for ideas for improving my fitness level.

Source: FITNESSGRAM Test Administration Manual, Second Edition

---

FITNESSGRAM

Personal Fitness Record

Name _____ School _____ Age ____ Grade ____ Ht ____ Wt ____

	Date:		Date:		Date:	
	Score	HFZ	Score	HFZ	Score	HFZ
Aerobic capacity:						
_____						
Curl-up						
Trunk lift						
Upper body strength:						
_____						
Flexibility:						
_____						
Skinfolds:						
Triceps						
Calf						
Total						

Note: HFZ indicates you have performed in the Healthy Fitness Zone.

I understand that my fitness record is personal. I do not have to share my results. My fitness record is important since it allows me to check my fitness level. If it is low, I will need to do more activity. If it is acceptable, I need to continue my current activity level. I know that I can ask my teacher for ideas for improving my fitness level.

Source: FITNESSGRAM Test Administration Manual, Second Edition

FITNESSGRAM

ACTIVITYGRAM Logging Chart

Name_____ Age____ Teacher_____ Grade____

Record the *primary* activity you did during each 30-minute interval during the day using the list at the bottom of the page. Then select an intensity level that best describes how it felt (Light: "Easy"; Moderate: "Not too tiring"; Vigorous: "Very tiring"). *Note:* All time periods of rest should have Rest checked for intensity level.

Time	Activity	Rest	Light	Mod.	Vig.	Time	Activity	Rest	Light	Mod.	Vig.
7:00						3:00					
7:30						3:30					
8:00						4:00					
8:30						4:30					
9:00						5:00					
9:30						5:30					
10:00						6:00					
10:30						6:30					
11:00						7:00					
11:30						7:30					
12:00						8:00					
12:30						8:30					
1:00						9:00					
1:30						9:30					
2:00						10:00					
2:30						10:30					

Categories of Physical Activities

Lifestyle activity	Active aerobics	Active sports	Muscle fitness activities	Flexibility exercises	Rest and inactivity
"Activities that I do as part of my normal day"	"Activities that I do for aerobic fitness"	"Activities that I do for sports and recreation"	"Activities that I do for muscular fitness"	"Activities that I do for flexibility and fun"	"Things I do when I am not active"
1. Walking, bicycling, or skateboarding	11. Aerobic dance activity	21. Field sports (baseball, softball, football, soccer, etc. . .)	31. Gymnastics or cheer, dance or drill teams	41. Martial arts (Tai Chi)	51. Schoolwork, homework or reading
2. Housework or yardwork	12. Aerobic gym equipment (stairclimber, treadmill, etc. . .)	22. Court sports (basketball, volleyball, soccer, hockey, etc. . .)	32. Track and field sports (jumping, throwing, etc. . .)	42. Stretching	52. Computer games or TV/videos
3. Playing active games or dancing	13. Aerobic activity (bicycling, running, skating, etc. . .)	23. Raquet sports (tennis, racquet-ball, etc. . .)	33. Weight lifting or calisthenics (pushups, situps, etc. . .)	43. Yoga	53. Eating or resting
4. Work—active job	14. Aerobic activity in physical education	24. Sports during physical education	34. Wrestling or Martial Arts (Karate, Aikido)	44. Ballet dancing	54. Sleeping
5. Other _____	15. Other _____	25. Other _____	35. Other _____	45. Other _____	55. Other _____

Source: FITNESSGRAM Test Administration Manual, Second Edition

What did I do yesterday? Sample *ACTIVITYGRAM* Log

Name_____ Age____ Teacher_____ Grade____

Think back to yesterday and try to remember what you did after you got home from school. Record the *primary* activity you did during each 30-minute interval using the list at the bottom of the page. Then select an intensity level that best describes how it felt (Light: "Easy"; Moderate: "Not too tiring"; Vigorous: "Very tiring"). *Note:* All time periods of rest should have Rest checked for intensity level.

		Activity numbers	Rest	Light	Moderate	Vigorous
Afternoon	**3:00**					
	3:30					
	4:00					
	4:30					
Supper	**5:00**					
	5:30					
	6:00					
	6:30					
Evening	**7:00**					
	7:30					
	8:00					
	8:30					

Categories of Physical Activities

Lifestyle activity	Active aerobics	Active sports	Muscle fitness activities	Flexibility exercises	Rest and inactivity
"Activities that I do as part of my normal day"	"Activities that I do for aerobic fitness"	"Activities that I do for sports and recreation"	"Activities that I do for muscular fitness"	"Activities that I do for flexibility and fun"	"Things I do when I am not active"
1. Walking, bicycling, or skateboarding	11. Aerobic dance activity	21. Field sports (baseball, softball, football, soccer, etc. . .)	31. Gymnastics or cheer, dance or drill teams	41. Martial arts (Tai Chi)	51. Schoolwork, homework or reading
2. Housework or yardwork	12. Aerobic gym equipment (stairclimber, treadmill, etc. . .)	22. Court sports (basketball, volleyball, soccer, hockey, etc. . .)	32. Track and field sports (jumping, throwing, etc. . .)	42. Stretching	52. Computer games or TV/ videos
3. Playing active games or dancing	13. Aerobic activity (bicycling, running, skating, etc. . .)	23. Raquet sports (tennis, racquet-ball, etc. . .)	33. Weight lifting or calisthenics (pushups, situps, etc. . .)	43. Yoga	53. Eating or resting
4. Work— active job	14. Aerobic activity in physical educa-tion	24. Sports during physical education	34. Wrestling or Martial Arts (Karate, Aikido)	44. Ballet dancing	54. Sleeping
5. Other _____	15. Other _____	25. Other _____	35. Other _____	45. Other _____	55. Other _____

Source: FITNESSGRAM Test Administration Manual, Second Edition

Appendix D

Health-Related Fitness Tracking Charts—Copy Masters

FITNESSGRAM®

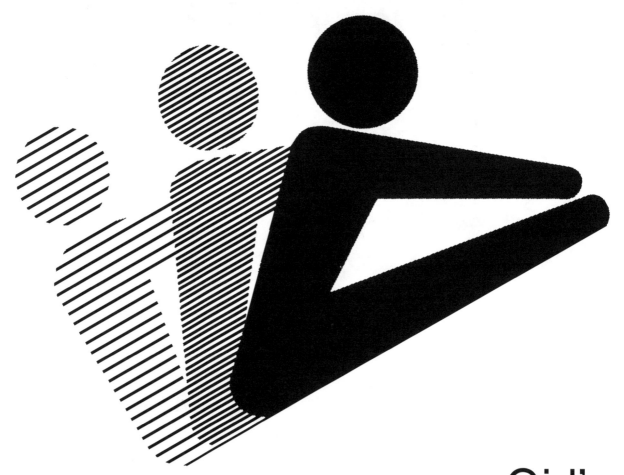

Girl's
Health-Related Fitness
Tracking Chart

_____   _____
Student   School District

FITNESSGRAM

How to Use

FITNESSGRAM Longitudinal Tracking Chart is to be used to chart the fitness level of each individual from the first *FITNESSGRAM* testing experience to the last. There is a graph for every test item to be used in plotting the scores each test date. The gray shaded area in the graph indicates the Healthy Fitness Zone for that test item. Use this chart in addition to the *FITNESSGRAM* to communicate long-term progress in maintaining healthy fitness levels.

Follow these simple instructions:

1. Write the child's name on the front of the chart in the space provided.

2. Mark the current score for each test on the appropriate graph. It is suggested that a distinctive mark that is easy to make such as a ■, ●, ✖ be used.

3. At the next test date, mark the score with the same symbol. Draw a line connecting the two marks.

4. Notice the minor mark is included on the X-axis indicating 6-month intervals to use if testing is conducted twice during a school year.

5. The graphs for height and weight indicate the 10th, 50th, and 95th percentile levels for growth.

Example:

Curl-Up

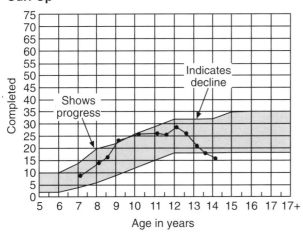

Other Suggestions

- Use the graphs to chart the progress for an entire school district by using the mean scores from the Statistical Summary Report. These reports can be produced with the *FITNESSGRAM* software program.

- Allow children to complete their own charts and integrate this activity into math class.

Aerobic Capacity

One-Mile Run/Walk

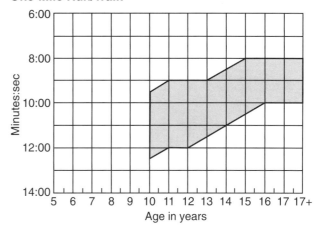

The PACER

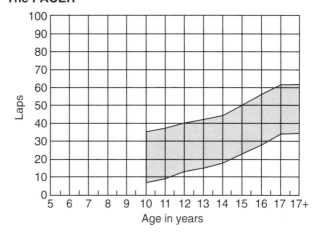

V̇O₂max

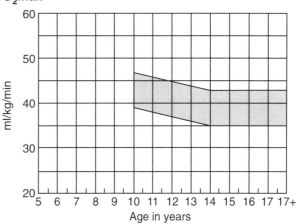

Body Size and Body Composition

Percent Body Fat
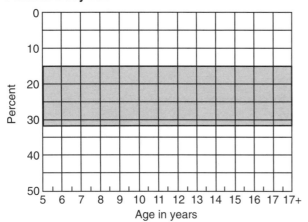

Body Mass Index
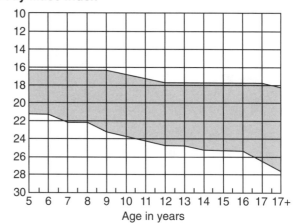

Height
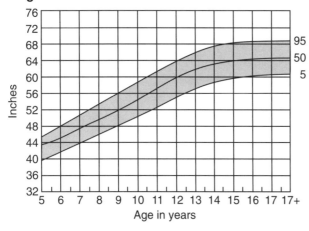

Weight
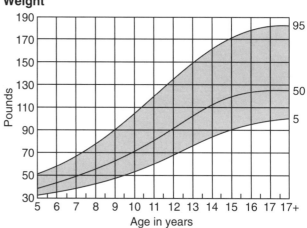

Muscle Strength, Endurance, and Flexibility

Curl-Up
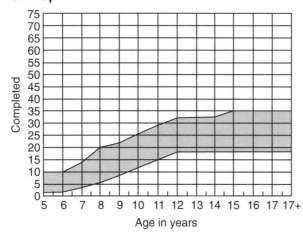

Trunk Lift
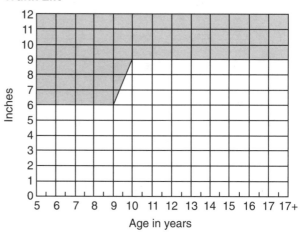

FITNESSGRAM

Muscle Strength, Endurance, and Flexibility

Push-Ups
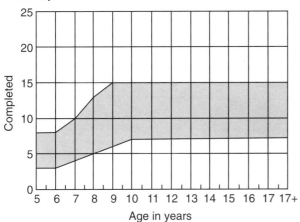

Modified Pull-Ups
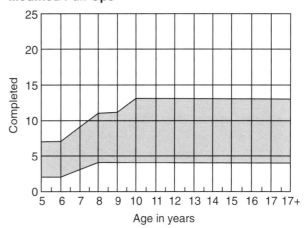

Pull-Ups
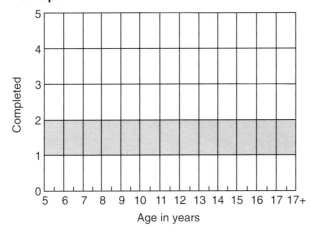

Flexed Arm Hang
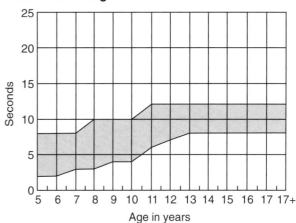

Back-Saver Sit and Reach
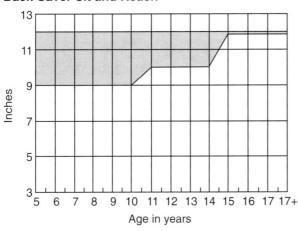

Right Side ■—■—■   Left Side ●—●—●

FITNESSGRAM®

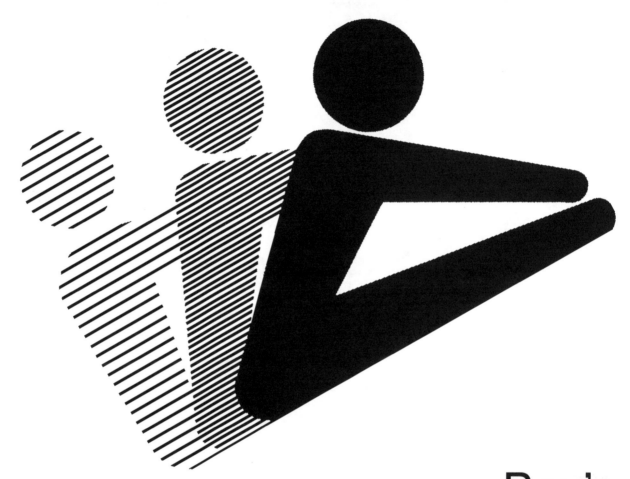

Boy's
Health-Related Fitness
Tracking Chart

| Student | School District |

How to Use

FITNESSGRAM Longitudinal Tracking Chart is to be used to chart the fitness level of each individual from the first *FITNESSGRAM* testing experience to the last. There is a graph for every test item to be used in plotting the scores each test date. The gray shaded area in the graph indicates the Healthy Fitness Zone for that test item. Use this chart in addition to the *FITNESSGRAM* to communicate long-term progress in maintaining healthy fitness levels.

Follow these simple instructions:

1. Write the child's name on the front of the chart in the space provided.
2. Mark the current score for each test on the appropriate graph. It is suggested that a distinctive mark that is easy to make such as a ■, ●, ✖ be used.
3. At the next test date, mark the score with the same symbol. Draw a line connecting the two marks.
4. Notice the minor mark is included on the X-axis indicating 6-month intervals to use if testing is conducted twice during a school year.
5. The graphs for height and weight indicate the 10th, 50th, and 95th percentile levels for growth.

Example:

Curl-Up

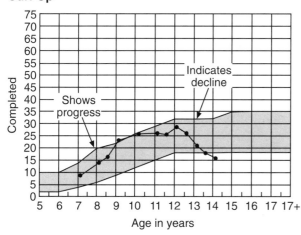

Other Suggestions

- Use the graphs to chart the progress for an entire school district by using the mean scores from the Statistical Summary Report. These reports can be produced with the *FITNESSGRAM* software program.
- Allow children to complete their own charts and integrate this activity into math class.

Aerobic Capacity

One-Mile Run/Walk

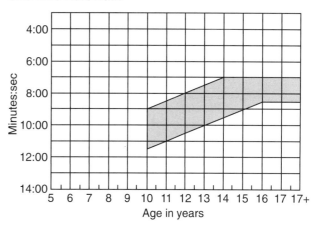

The PACER

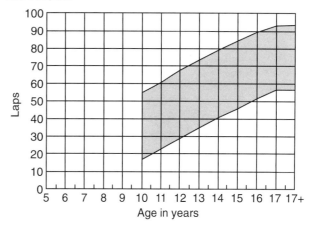

V̇O₂max

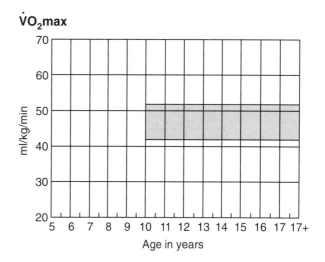

Body Size and Body Composition

Percent Body Fat

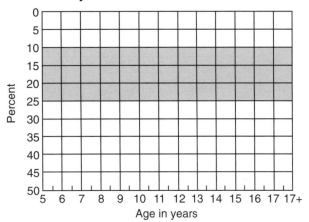

Body Mass Index

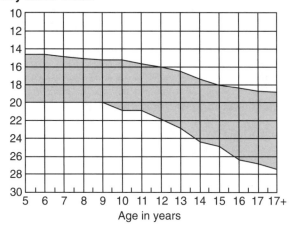

Height

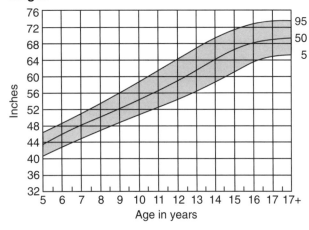

Weight

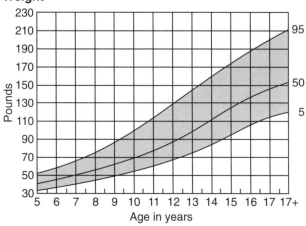

Muscle Strength, Endurance, and Flexibility

Curl-Up

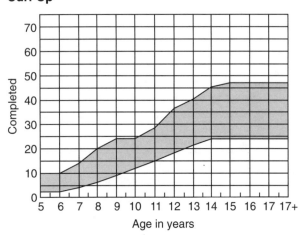

Trunk Lift

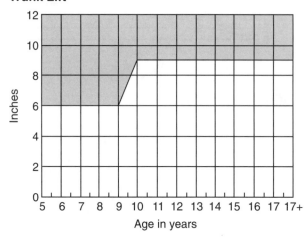

Muscle Strength, Endurance, and Flexibility

Push-Ups

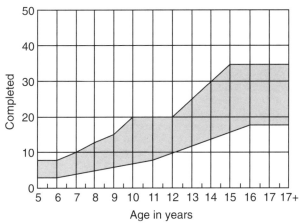

Modified Pull-Ups

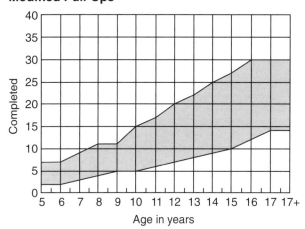

Pull-Ups

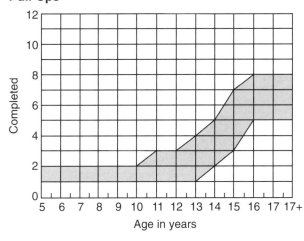

Flexed Arm Hang

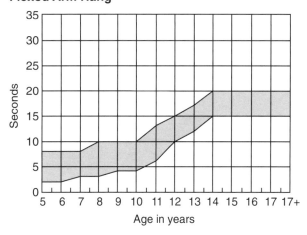

Back-Saver Sit and Reach

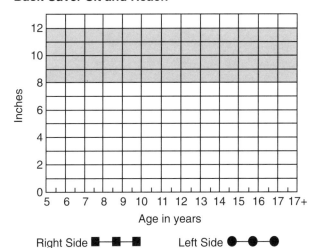

Right Side ■─■─■   Left Side ●─●─●

Appendix E
Software User Manual

Contents

System Requirements

Windows

- Windows 9x/NT 4.0 workstation
- 486 or higher
- at least 16 MB; 32 MG recommended
- color monitor
- 3.5 floppy disk or CD-ROM drive
- Settings to 800 x 600 screen resolution or higher

Macintosh

- Power Mac recommended
- System 7.x or higher
- at least 16 MB; 32 MG recommended
- color monitor
- 3.5 floppy disk or CD-ROM drive
- Settings to 832 x 624 screen resolution or higher

Please follow the steps listed below to install your *FITNESSGRAM* software to either a Windows or Macintosh computer. *Do not install FITNESSGRAM to a network drive. Instead, install the program to your hard drive, then create one or more databases on a network drive to run FITNESSGRAM on a network.* See page 109 for information on creating a database to a network drive. After installation and before you can begin working in *FITNESSGRAM*, you'll need to configure your software by obtaining an unlock code. Those procedures are listed after the installation instructions.

Installation of *FITNESSGRAM* for Windows

From disk (teacher program only)

1. Insert disk 1 into the floppy drive.
2. Click on the "Start" button on your toolbar in the lower left-hand corner of the screen. Then select the "Run..." icon.
3. In the text box type "a:\setup.exe" or "b:\setup.exe". (Use the letter that corresponds to your floppy drive). Click OK.
4. Follow the prompts to install the software. Remember to install *FITNESSGRAM* to your hard drive, not to a network drive.
5. The default file path is c:\ftgr60.
6. Display settings to 800 x 600 or higher screen resolution.

From CD

The CD includes both the teacher and student *FITNESSGRAM* programs. During the install process you'll need to select whether to install either the teacher or student program or to install both programs. The install process is the same regardless of your selection.

1. Insert the *FITNESSGRAM* CD-ROM into the drive.
2. Click on the "Start" button on your toolbar in the lower left hand corner of the screen. Then select the "Run..." icon.
3. In the text box type "x:\setup.exe" (X is the letter that corresponds to your CD-ROM drive). Click OK.
4. Follow the prompts to install the software. Remember, install *FITNESSGRAM* to your hard drive, not to a network drive.
5. The default file path is c:\ftgr60.
6. Display settings to 800 x 600 or higher screen resolution.

Installation of *FITNESSGRAM* for Macintosh

From disk (teacher program only)

1. Insert disk 1 into the floppy drive.
2. Double click the icon FITNESSGRAM6 located on your desktop.
3. Double click on the file FITNESSGRAM Installer to begin the installation.
4. Follow the prompts to install the software. Remember to install *FITNESSGRAM* to your hard drive, not to a network drive.
5. The default folder name is ftgr60.
6. Settings should be set to 832 x 624 screen resolution or higher.

From CD

The CD includes both the teacher and student *FITNESSGRAM* programs. During the install process you'll need to select whether to install either the teacher or student program or both programs. The install process is the same regardless of your selection.

1. Insert the *FITNESSGRAM* CD-ROM into the drive.
2. Double click the icon FITNESSGRAM6 located on your desktop.

3. Double click on the file FITNESSGRAM Installer to begin the installation.

4. Follow the prompts to install the software. Remember to install *FITNESSGRAM* to your hard drive, not to a network drive.

5. The default folder name is ftgr60.

6. Settings should be set to 832 x 624 screen resolution or higher.

Running *FITNESSGRAM* on a Network

FITNESSGRAM databases can be created on any network drive. For any user to be able to use a database on a network drive, that user must have the read/write permission to the network drive and folder where the database is located. If necessary, your network administrator will have to modify the read/write permission. Follow these steps to ensure correct network use of *FITNESSGRAM*.

1. To run *FITNESSGRAM* on a network, your first step is to install the teacher program to your hard drive.

2. Create one or more teacher databases on a network drive (see page 109).

3. If you have the student *FITNESSGRAM*, then you will need to install it on all workstations (only hard drives) to be used by your students.

4. Direct or 'point' the student program to the correct teacher database. See page 111 for complete information on using the student *FITNESSGRAM*.

FITNESSGRAM Configuration

When you use the Teacher program for the first time (after installation), you will see a message telling you to configure your program. When you click OK, a dialog box appears asking you to type in your unlock code, city name, and school name. The unlock code is part of the security of *FITNESSGRAM* and allows you to use the software.

Here's what you need to do in order to obtain your unlock code.

1. To receive your unlock code, please contact Human Kinetics Customer Service at 1-800-747-4457 between 8 A.M. and 5 P.M. (CST), Monday through Friday. If you purchased the software outside the United States, please contact the HK Subsidiary you

purchased the software from. The sticker on the outside of the shrinkwrap will help you determine which subsidiary to contact.

HK Australia: (08) 82771555 (9 A.M. - 5 P.M.)

HK Canada: 1-800-465-7301 (9 A.M. - 5 P.M.) (EST)

HK Europe: +44 (0) 113-278 1708
(8.30 A.M. – 5.30 P.M.)

HK New Zealand: 09-523-3462 (8 A.M. - 5 P.M.)

2. The customer service representative will confirm your order and ask for your CITY NAME and SCHOOL NAME. Please write down this information as you will need to enter it on the configuration screen; it must be an exact match. The school name is used on all *FITNESSGRAM* reports.

3. You will be given an unlock code. Please write down this code as well as you will need to enter it in the configuration screen; it must be an exact match. Keep your unlock code and other information in a safe place in case you need to refer to it later.

4. On the configuration screen, type in your unlock code, city name, school name, and other optional information such as School ID, District Name, and District ID. Write down this information and keep with the unlock code in case you need to refer to it later.

5. Request Ethnicity Information. Some schools need to report this information to state and local agencies. Click the checkbox if you would like this field to appear in the My Info section of the student software (see page 118). Note: This field also appears in the teacher section of the software.

6. If you would like to add more schools to this installation of *FITNESSGRAM*, then click the Add button. You will need to contact Human Kinetics Customer Service for an unlock code for each school you want to add. When your order has been confirmed, you will be given an additional unlock code(s).

7. Click OK when finished.

8. You are now able to use *FITNESSGRAM*.

Teacher *FITNESSGRAM*

It's easy to move around in *FITNESSGRAM* and to get from one screen to another (i.e., entering information, viewing reports, creating tests, etc.). Primary program features are accessible through the four buttons on the left side of the main screen with reports and administrative functions accessed via the pull-down menus located at the top of each screen.

Main Screen

There are four data entry functions on the main screen:

1. **Teachers:** Enter names of all teachers using *FITNESSGRAM.*
2. **Classes:** Enter names of classes for each teacher. Each teacher is linked to one or more classes.
3. **Students:** Enter names and demographic information for each student. Students are linked to a specific teacher and class.
4. **Tests:** Enter test names and dates, then enter fitness test scores for your students. Tests are also linked to a specific teacher and class.

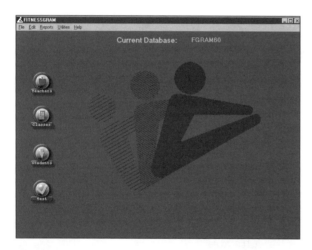

Main screen.

Pull-Down Menus

File Menu
- **New and Open:** These two options are used to create a new or open an existing database containing teacher, class, student, and test information. See page 109.
- **Export/Import:** *FITNESSGRAM* offers several options for importing and exporting student and test information. See page 113 for options and instructions.
- **Exit**

Edit Menu
- In this menu you'll find standard Windows or Macintosh commands such as Undo, Cut, Copy, and Paste.

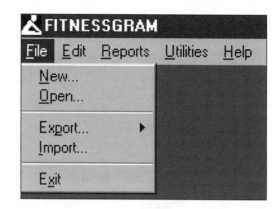

File pull-down menu (Windows®).

Reports Menu
- Use this feature to create a variety of reports for yourself and to print the *FITNESSGRAM* report for your students and parents. See page 113 for more information.

Utilities Menu
- The options listed in this menu deal with administrative tasks such as year-end processing, promoting students to the next grade level, moving students to new classes, deleting selected or all data, database maintenance, and data backup. See pages 115-117 for more information.

Help Menu
- Takes you to an extensive Help file.

Getting Started

Before you can enter students and test scores, you need to enter teacher and class information. This can be done manually or you can use the import utility to get student data into the computer from other databases such as your grading or attendance programs, or from an earlier version of the software (FitnessGram 5.0). See page 114 for import options.

To begin:
- Windows users go to the Start Menu. Select Programs, FITNESSGRAM, then click on Teacher Edition.
- Macintosh users go to the ftgr60 folder and click on Teacher Edition.

Follow these easy steps to setting up *FITNESSGRAM.*

1. Create a database to store teacher, class, student, and test information. If you prefer, you can use the *FITNESSGRAM* FGRAM60 data-

base to store your information. This is a blank database already created for you. Databases can be created on your hard drive or on a network drive.

2. Enter teacher information for all teachers using *FITNESSGRAM*.

3. Enter class information for each teacher.

4. Enter student information.

5. Enter test events.

6. Enter test scores for each student.

7. Print a variety of reports, including the *FITNESSGRAM* report for students and parents.

If you installed the student application of *FITNESSGRAM*, you can have your students enter their own test scores. See page 117 for information on Student *FITNESSGRAM*.

Working With Databases

The *FITNESSGRAM* database stores teacher, class, student, and test information. A database can include many records so one database may be sufficient for your needs. However, after you have had a chance to look at *FITNESSGRAM*, you may decide to create separate databases for all teachers using *FITNESSGRAM* or you may want to create separate databases for different grades. Take a look at the Sample database and see how it is structured, then decide if you need more than one database for you and your school. A blank database, FGRAM60, has already been created for you.

Create a New Database

You can create databases on your hard drive or on a network drive.

- Click the File pull-down menu, then click New.
- Using the Browse button, select the location for the new database. The default file path for Windows users is c:\ftgr60\teacher. For Macintosh users, the default location is the ftgr60 folder.
- A database can be created on your hard drive or on a network drive.
- Enter the new database name and Click OK.
- This will add the new database to *FITNESSGRAM*.

Open a Database

- A blank database, FGRAM60 has already been created for you.

- Click the File pull-down menu, then click Open.
- Using the Browse button, select the desired database from the list box. The default file path for Windows users is c:\ftgr60\teacher. For Macintosh users, the default location is the ftgr60 folder, then select teacher. This is where the Sample and FGRAM60 databases are located. Remember that a database can be created anywhere on your hard drive or on a network drive.
- Click OK when the database has been selected.

Delete a Database

- You can't delete a database from within *FITNESSGRAM*, but you can delete information from the database. See page 110 for instructions on deleting data.

 # Working With Teachers

In *FITNESSGRAM*, all aspects of the program—classes, students, and tests—are tied to a teacher's name. A teacher can have more than one class and one test just as a class can have more than one test assigned to it (i.e., Fall Fitness Test and Spring Fitness Test). In Teachers, you can add new teachers, edit current teacher information, and delete teachers from the database.

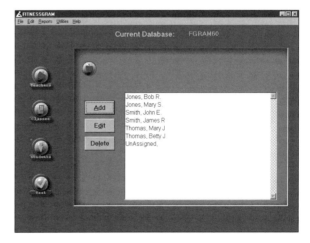

Teacher menu.

Add a Teacher

- First step is to add the names of the Teachers who are using *FITNESSGRAM*. To access, click the Teachers button, then the Add button.
- At the pop-up box, enter the teacher's last name and first name. If there are teachers with

the same name using the program, then include a middle name or initial.

- When you are finished adding a teacher, click the OK button.
- When all teachers have been added, click the Cancel button.

Edit a Teacher

- To edit a teacher, highlight the teacher's name and click the Edit button.
- Make the necessary corrections and click OK when you are finished.

Delete a Teacher

- To delete a teacher from *FITNESSGRAM*, highlight the teacher's name and press the Delete button.
- *FITNESSGRAM* will verify if you do want to delete that teacher from the program. If so, press the Yes button or No to discontinue this action.

Unassigned Teacher

- Notice that one of the entries in Teachers is Unassigned. The Unassigned teacher cannot be deleted. You may have students who (for one reason or another) are not affiliated with a teacher. This student may have just moved in to the school district or may have been transferred to another teacher or it may be the end of the year and one or more students have not been assigned a teacher for the next school year. The Unassigned teacher is where these students are placed.
- If a teacher with classes and students is deleted, the students will automatically be assigned to the Unassigned teacher and class.

Notes

For information on moving students to new teachers or classes, including Unassigned, see page 116.

 Working With Classes

The second step is to add one or more classes to each teacher. Be descriptive in naming the class such as identifying each class by a teacher name or by a particular day and time or semester. To add, edit, or delete a class, click the Classes button.

Add a Class

- To add classes to teachers, click the Classes button.

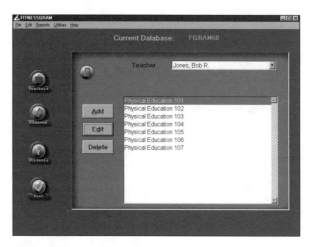

Classes menu.

- Select a teacher from the drop-down list then click the Add button.
- At the pop-up box, enter the name of the class. Click the OK button.
- Repeat for all classes using *FITNESSGRAM*.

Edit a Class

- To edit a class, click the Classes button.
- Choose a teacher from the drop-down list.
- Highlight the class you want to edit, then click the Edit button.
- Make the necessary corrections and click OK when finished.

Delete a Class

- To delete a class, click the Classes button.
- Choose a teacher from the drop-down list. Click the Add button.
- Highlight the class you want to delete, then click the Delete button.
- *FITNESSGRAM* will verify if you do want to delete the class from the database. If so, press the Yes button or No to discontinue this action.

Unassigned Class

- Notice that one of the entries in Classes is Unassigned. The Unassigned class is affiliated with the Unassigned Teacher. You cannot delete either of the Unassigned entries. Sometimes in the course of the school year, there may be students who (for one reason or another) are not affiliated with a class. This student may have just moved in to the school district or may have been transferred to or from another class or it may be the end of the year and one or more students have not been assigned a class. The Unassigned teacher and classes is where these students are placed.

- If a teacher with classes and students is deleted, the students will automatically be assigned to the Unassigned teacher and class.

Notes

For information on moving students to new classes, including Unassigned, see page 116.

 Working With Students

The third step is to add students to a particular teacher and class. Click the Students button to add, edit, or delete one or more students. Use the pull-down lists to select the teacher and class associated with a group of students.

Add a Student

- Select the right teacher and class from the pull-down lists.
- To add a student, click the Add button.
- When complete, click the OK button to add the student. To close the student information window, click the Cancel button.

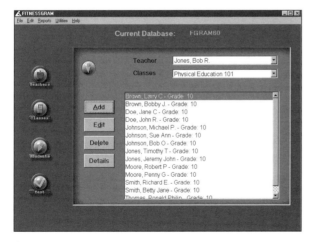

Student menu.

Notes

- A screen appears with a number of information fields. Required fields are marked with an *: last name and first name.

- Body Composition: If you have students who do not want to have body composition information (height, weight, percent body fat, BMI) printed on the *FITNESSGRAM* report, make sure the check box marked "Print Body Composition" is blank.

- If you do not assign a Student Number or ID to a student, *FITNESSGRAM* will automatically assign a number.

- The Ethnicity field is optional. It is included in *FITNESSGRAM* because some states must report this information to local or state agencies.

- If you are using the student *FITNESSGRAM,* then enter only the student's first name, last name, and password. You can either provide unique passwords for your students or automatically generate passwords for them. The student will enter the remaining information in the My Info screen of the student software. Note: Students can change their password in the My Info screen.

Entering Student Passwords

The Password field is used in the student application of *FITNESSGRAM*. There are two ways to assign passwords to students:

1. As you add students, type in a unique password for each.
2. After you enter student information, go into the student spreadsheet (via the Details button) to automatically generate passwords. Click the Generate Passwords button at the bottom of the screen. This utility will not overwrite passwords already entered for the student. You can print a report providing you with the students' names and passwords. See Reports page 113.

Student information spreadsheet.

Edit a Student

- Select the teacher and class from the pull-down lists.
- To edit a student name, highlight the student's name and click the Edit button.
- Make the necessary corrections and click OK when you are finished.
- Or click the Details button to make the corrections from the student spreadsheet.

Delete a Student

- Select the teacher and class from the pull-down lists.
- To delete a student, highlight the student's name and press the Delete button.
- *FITNESSGRAM* will verify that you do want to delete the student from the program. If so, press the Yes button or No to discontinue this action.

Notes

- To save time, you can import student information from a variety of databases. See page 114 for complete import information.
- See page 116 for information on assigning students to new classes or teachers, year-end processing of students, etc.
- Inactive/Active Student Status—When you add a student, *FITNESSGRAM* assumes that the student is "Active" until you change the status to Inactive. To change a student's status from Active to Inactive, click the Edit button. Click the check box if the student is Inactive. Notice that the student has been removed from your class. To change a student's status from inactive to active, see page 115.

 ## Working With Tests and Scores

The next step is to enter a *FITNESSGRAM* test event name and date. Finally, you enter test scores for your students. To add, edit, or delete test names, first select a teacher and class from the pull-down lists.

Add a Test

- Click the Test button. Then select the right teacher and class from the pull-down lists.
- To add a test event, click the Add button.
- Name the test event, then enter the date. Be sure to be descriptive in your test event names such as Spring 1999 or Grade 4 Fall '99 test. Do not use the individual names of test items (i.e., PACER, Push-up, etc.) to name a test event.

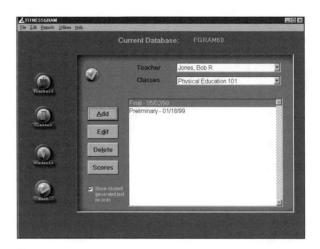

Test menu.

- When you are finished adding a test name and date, click the OK button.

Edit a Test

- To edit a test name, highlight the test you want to edit, then click on the Edit button.
- Make the necessary corrections and click OK when you are finished.

Delete a Test

- To delete a Test from *FITNESSGRAM*, highlight the test name, then press the Delete button.
- *FITNESSGRAM* will verify that you do want to delete the test from the program. If so, press the Yes button or No to discontinue this action.

Entering Test Scores

Press the Scores button to enter fitness test scores for your students. Use the Tab or Enter/return keys or your mouse to move from field to field. Highlight the field, then enter the test score.

Fullname	Ht(ft)	Ht(in)	Weight(lbs)	Pacer	Mile Run(Mi	Mile Run(Se	Walk Test(Mi	Walk Test(Se	Walk Test(He	Pushup	P
Brown, Bobby J.	5	11	168	20	7	25	15	26		10	5
Brown, Larry C	5	10	167	20	8	15	16	15		25	1
Doe, Jane C	5	04	123	30	8	16	18	18		20	5
Doe, John R.	5	09	151	20	7	2	15	17		5	8
Johnson, Bob O.	5	08	134	10	6	15	14	6		35	5
Johnson, Michael P.	6	02	141	5	10	25	25	28		20	1
Johnson, Sue Ann	5	01	105	11	12	36	32	35		25	5
Jones, Jeremy John	5	06	133	13	10	18	21	41		18	2
Jones, Timothy T	5	05	126	20	9	33	19	52		10	5
Moore, Penny O	5	08	126	30	7	18	15	9		6	3
Moore, Robert P	5	09	185	15	25	25	38	18		5	5
Smith, Betty Jane	5	07	150	13	7	18	16	32		4	7
Smith, Richard E.	5	10	190	15	16	22	32	45		15	5
Thomas, Ronald Phil	6	03	225	25	7	35	16	42		60	1

Student test scores screen.

Notes

- If you prefer, you can print a score sheet to enter test scores on paper then transfer to the software at a later date. Click the Scores button. At the bottom of the screen, click the Print Score Sheet button.

- If you have students who do not want to have body composition information (height, weight, percent body fat, BMI) printed on the *FITNESSGRAM* report, make sure the check box marked "Print Body Composition" in the Add or Edit Student screens is blank.

- If you installed student *FITNESSGRAM*, then students can generate their own tests. By clicking the check box next to Show Student Generated Test Records, student generated tests will automatically be displayed onscreen.

- A *FITNESSGRAM* report can also be printed from the Test function.

Reports

A variety of reports are available from the *FITNESSGRAM* software.

- Go to the Reports pull-down menu and select Reports. A pop-up screen appears with report options.

- Select the name of the teacher followed by the class name.

- Notice that on the right side of the screen, there are two types of reports—Student Reports and Test Date Reports.

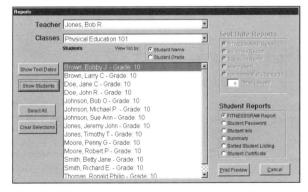

Reports screen.

Student Reports

To select Student Reports, press the Show Students button. Further select reports by choosing either the view list by Student Name or Student Grade.

- **Report for a single student**. If you want to see a report for a single student, then highlight the student name and select the type of report to view or print.

- **Report for more than one student.** If you want to see a report for more than one student, then highlight the student name and press the Ctrl key simultaneously.

- **Report for all students.** If you want to see a report for all the students in the test date, then press the Select All button.

To clear your selections, press the Clear Selections button.

Student Report Options

- *FITNESSGRAM* **Report**–This report is for students and parents. It displays the student's fitness test scores, the relationship of the scores to the Healthy Fitness Zone, and information on how to improve or maintain current fitness levels. Before printing, you'll see several options for printing the *FITNESSGRAM* report. You can choose to print all reports or the most recent *FITNESSGRAM* report for the selected student(s), or print the reports on plain paper or use preprinted test forms, or print the *FITNESSGRAM* information page (the reverse side of the report). Once you have made your selections, press OK.

- **Student Password** – Report listing students' name, ID, and passwords.

- **Student Info** – Report listing of students' name, ID, birthdate, nickname, gender, and grade.

- **Summary Report** - This report prints a summary of test results.

- **Sorted Student Listing** - This menu item prints a report sorted by student's last name or by grade. The report provides the student ID and a list of the test events the student has in the current database.

- **Student Certificate** – This menu item generates a recognition certificate for selected students that can be personalized by name and achievement.

Select the report option and press the Print Preview button. To print, press the printer icon.

Test Date Reports

To select Test Date Reports, press the Show Test Dates button.

- **Report for single test.** If you want to see a report for a single test, then highlight the test name and select the type of report to view or print.

- **Report for more than one test.** If you want to see a report for more than one test, then highlight the test name and press the Ctrl key simultaneously.
- **Report for all tests.** If you want to see a report for all the tests for that particular teacher and class, then press the Select All button.

To clear your selections, press the Clear Selections button.

Test Date Report Options

- *FITNESSGRAM* **Report** — This is the same report as listed under Student Report options.
- **Summary Report** — This report prints a summary of test results.
- **Statistical Report** — This statistical summary report contains group summary information including mean, standard deviation, range of scores and percentage of students achieving the Healthy Fitness Zone. This report is printed by test item, gender, and age.
- **Score Sheet** — This menu item prints a score sheet of the students' test scores for the selected test date. For a blank score sheet that you can use to record scores and then transfer them to the software at a later date, see page 113.
- **Achievement of Standards** — This menu item prints a listing of students achieving the Healthy Fitness Zone for a specified number of test items on a specific test date.

Select the report option and press the Print Preview button. To print, press the printer icon.

Import/Export Options

The *FITNESSGRAM* import and export features allow you to transfer data between a variety of sources. With the import features, you can save yourself time by not having to manually enter the same student information. Several options are listed here. Please see the Help files for step-by-step instructions.

To access the Export and Import functions, select Import or Export from the File pull-down menu.

Import Options

- *FITNESSGRAM* **6.0 Format** — Automatically import data exported from other *FITNESSGRAM* 6.0 databases using the default *FITNESSGRAM* 6.0 format.

- **FitnessGram 5.0 Import** — Still using the previous version of FitnessGram? This option allows you to automatically convert information exported from a FitnessGram 5.0 database.
- **Custom** — This option allows you to specify the variables, variable order, and the format for any date fields.
- **Scanned Data** — With this option, you import scanned data that was created using scanning software. Some scanning software includes appropriate form and definition files. These files are *not* included with *FITNESSGRAM.*
- **American Fitness Alliance Default** — This option allows you to only import student information (not test results) from other software programs available from the American Fitness Alliance such as FitSmart and Fitness Challenge.

After you select the import option, you need to indicate the file pathway and that the data be imported into the Unassigned teacher and class. To move students from Unassigned, see page 116.

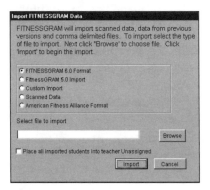

Import menu.

Export Options

- *FITNESSGRAM* **6.0 Default** – Automatically exports all *FITNESSGRAM* data in a standard format. You will then be able to automatically import the same data into another *FITNESSGRAM* 6.0 database.
- **Custom** – With this option, you specify the variables and file format for the exported data by marking the appropriate check box.
- **American Fitness Alliance Default** – This option allows you to export information in a format that can automatically be imported into other software programs available from the American Fitness Alliance such as FitSmart and Fitness Challenge.

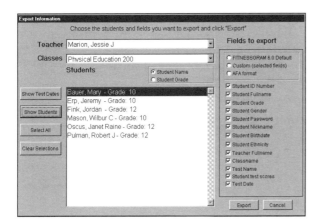

Export menu.

General export instructions:

- When you select Export from the File pull-down menu, you will need to select either *FITNESSGRAM* data or *ACTIVITYGRAM* data. Several options are available to export information from *FITNESSGRAM.*
- Notice that the *FITNESSGRAM* export screen is similar to the Report screen. You will first need to select the appropriate teacher and class from the pull-down lists. With all *FITNESSGRAM* export options, you will be able to further select by test date(s) or by student(s).
- On the right side of the screen, select the type of export. Once you have made your selections, press the Export button.
- Indicate which *FITNESSGRAM* to export–all *FITNESSGRAMS* or the most recent.
- The last step is to select the file type. Several file types are listed. Press the OK button to export data.
- If planning to import data back into *FITNESSGRAM,* you should select the *FITNESSGRAM* 6.0 default file format.

Please read the Help files for additional information on exporting data.

ACTIVITYGRAM Export

- To export *ACTIVTYGRAM* Data, select *ACTVITYGRAM* data from the Export option.
- Specify the file type for the export. Press OK to export data.
- At the Save As screen, select the file path to save the data. The default file name is atgexport. It will be saved as a text file. Press the Save button.

- The *ACTIVITYGRAM* export is available to facilitate the return of research data.

Administrative Functions

To access the administrative functions of *FITNESSGRAM,* use the Utilities pull-down menu and select one of the following:

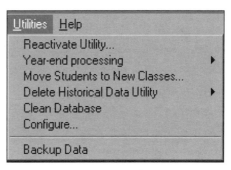

Utilities menu (Windows®).

1. Reactivate Utility
2. Year-end Processing–Consists of two options: Promote Students and Move Students to New Classes
3. Move Students to New Classes
4. Delete Historical Data Utility–Consists of two options: Delete Selected Data and Delete All Data.
5. Clean Database
6. Configure
7. Backup Data

Basic information is listed in this manual. For step-by-step instructions, please read the Help files.

Reactivate Utility

To change a student's status from inactive to active, go to the Utilities pull-down menu and select Reactivate Utility. Highlight the name of the student and press the Reactivate button. The student is now placed in the Unassigned Teacher and Class. To move the student from Unassigned to a teacher and class, see Moving Students to New Classes.

Year End Processing

From this option, select either Promoting Students or Move Students to New Classes and Teachers.

Promote Students

This selection will promote all the students in the *FITNESSGRAM* database one grade level and remove all class assignments. The students will be moved to the "Unassigned" teacher and class.

Note: *FITNESSGRAM* will inform you when the promote feature was last used. You should *only* promote students once during a school year. If the feature has already been used this school year, do not use it again.

- If you are uncertain whether you should run this utility, click the No button. Verify the grade levels of students in the database before running again.
- Click the Yes button to promote students and clear class assignments.

Move Students to New Classes (and Teachers)

- Select the current teacher and class location for the student(s) from the "Move Students From" drop-down lists. Generally, students needing to be assigned to a new class are in the "Unassigned" teacher and class.
- Select the new teacher and the class location for the student(s) from the "Move Students To" drop-down lists.
- Select the student(s) from the list box on the left (move from) box and Click on the right arrow which moves student to the new teacher and class assignment (move to) box.
- Click on OK when you have assigned all desired students to a new teacher and class.

Move Students to New Classes

- From this option, select the current teacher and class location for the student(s) from the Move Students from drop-down list. Generally, students needing to be assigned to a new class are in the "Unassigned" teacher and class.
- Select the new teacher and the class location for the student(s) from the "Move Students To" drop-down list.
- Select the student(s) from the list box on the left (move from) box and click on the right arrow which moves student to the new teacher and class assignment (move to) box.
- Click on OK when you have assigned all desired students to a new teacher and class.

Delete Historical Data Utility

The delete utility allows you to delete *FITNESSGRAM* data using two methods: by select-

ing specific data and by deleting all data in the open database. Use this utility carefully. If you are unsure as to the consequences of deleting *FITNESSGRAM* data, then it is recommended you make a backup of the database for future reference. See page 117 for information on backup.

Delete Selected Data

- To select, click the circle next to the item(s) you want to delete.
- If required, enter the years or grades of items that will be deleted.
- Click on Delete button. You will be asked to confirm the deletion. Click Yes if you wish to continue with the deletion of the data. Click No if you wish to cancel the deletion.

Delete All Data

This option deletes all data from the open database, so use this item very carefully. You might prefer to simply create a new database under the File pull-down menu. If you are running short of hard disk space, you can move the old database directory to a floppy or zip disk. Before you attempt to move the database directory to a disk, run Clean Database from the Utilities pull-down menu.

- Click Yes if you wish to continue the deletion of data.
- Click No if you wish to cancel the deletion.

Clean Database

Use this utility to periodically "purge" deleted data from your database. If your database has become excessively large and you have been routinely deleting information, *Clean Database* will actually remove all of the deleted information from the database and reduce its size.

- Click Yes if you wish to continue the clean routine.
- Click No if you wish to cancel the clean routine.

Configure *FITNESSGRAM*

You won't be able to modify any of the configuration information entered during the installation process. However, you can select or de-select the Request Ethnicity Information box at any time. This gives you the option of having this field appear in the My Info screen of the student program. If you do not want this information displayed in the student *FITNESSGRAM*, then make sure this box is left blank.

Backup Data

This utility will allow you to make a backup of the currently selected *FITNESSGRAM* data directory.

- Click on the Browse button to select the destination drive and directory for the backup. (The directory that is currently active in *FITNESSGRAM* is the source directory for the backup operation.) Make sure you do not copy over an existing database.
- Click OK to start the backup process.
- When the backup is completed, the opening window of *FITNESSGRAM* is displayed.

Backup data can be restored to your hard drive by copying the backup directory to the FTGR60/teacher directory.

Student *FITNESSGRAM*

- The student software will need to be installed on the hard drives of all workstations used by students.
- Make sure the settings for each computer are correct for screen resolution.
- In order to use the program, the Student software has to be 'pointed' or directed to the right database in the Teacher *FITNESSGRAM*.
- Windows users go to the Start Menu. Select Programs, *FITNESSGRAM,* then click on Student Edition.
- Macintosh users go to the ftgr60 folder and click on Student Edition.
- At the Student log-on screen. Type in *FITNESSGRAM* in all three fields—first name, last name, and password.
- A dialog box appears displaying the various drives and databases. Using the Browse button, select the appropriate drive where the database is located, then highlight the database you wish to use for Student *FITNESSGRAM*. Click OK.
- You will need to follow this procedure for each workstation.
- To start the student program, click Student Edition again.
- The log-on screen will reappear. Instruct the students to type in their first name, last name, and password.

How Students Log On

At the log-on screen, instruct your students to enter their first and last names, then their passwords. Click the Log-in Now button.

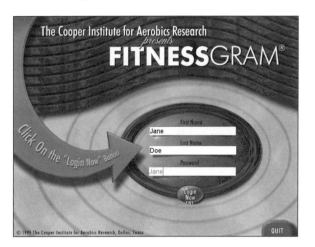

Student log-on screen.

Navigation Buttons

Have your students look for these navigation buttons throughout the student program.

- View or Print a Report–Students can instantly see or print a report on their progress.
- Main Menu—Takes the student back to the *FITNESSGRAM* Main Menu.
- Quit—Exits the program.

Main Menu Screen

At the main menu screen, instruct your students to click on either *FITNESSGRAM* to record test scores and take the physical activity questionnaire or the *ACTIVITYGRAM* to record their fitness activities for a two or three day period.

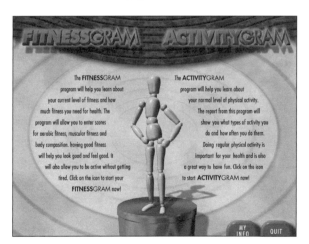

Main Menu screen.

My Info

In My Info, students enter or verify (if entered in the Teacher software) several pieces of information, including

- Nickname
- Gender
- Birthdate
- Grade
- Password (students can change a previously entered password)
- Short description—This is the ethnicity box that is also present in the Teacher *FITNESSGRAM*. If you do not want this field displayed, then you will need to go into the Utilities pull-down menu and select Configure. Make sure the Request Ethnicity Information check box is blank.

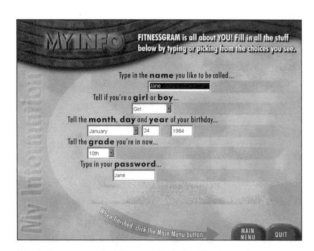

My Info screen (without ethnicity displayed).

FITNESSGRAM

Access *FITNESSGRAM* from the Main Menu.

1. To start a new *FITNESSGRAM* for yourself, click the New icon.
2. To Look over, Change, or Add to an existing *FITNESSGRAM*, select the *FITNESSGRAM* from the list, then click the Open icon.
3. To Remove a *FITNESSGRAM* from the list, select the *FITNESSGRAM*, then press the Delete icon.

Entering Fitness Test Scores

- Click the Scores button to enter test scores.
- Tell your students to follow the on-screen instructions for entering information for each

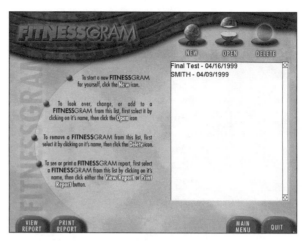

FITNESSGRAM menu screen.

test. (Note: It's best to review the instructions before having your students enter their test scores.)

- To access a specific test, simply click on the test name or data field, and enter the appropriate score in the boxes located at the top of the screen.
- Click the I'm Done button or Enter key. The test score will be displayed with the test.

To correct an entry, tell your students to click on the appropriate test button and reenter the test score.

To delete an entry, click on the appropriate test button, highlight the score, and press the I'm Done button.

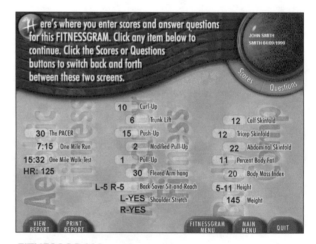

FITNESSGRAM scores screen.

Physical Activity Questionnaire

In this portion of the Student *FITNESSGRAM*, have your students enter the number of days during the last seven days they participate in aerobic, strength, and flexibility activities.

- Click the Questions button to access the questionnaire.
- Have the students click on the activity type.
- Read the question and instructions at the top of the screen and select the number of days in the text box.
- Click the I'm Done button when finished.
- The number of days spent in an activity will be reflected in the student's *FITNESSGRAM* report.

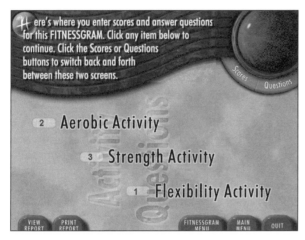

Questionnaire screen.

View or Print a *FITNESSGRAM* Report

Students view results of their fitness scores via the *FITNESSGRAM* report. Also printed are recommendations for improving fitness levels. This is the same report that is printed from the Teacher software. See page 35 for an example of this report.

ACTIVITYGRAM

In the *ACTIVITYGRAM*, students provide information on their daily activities for a two or three day period. This information is then compiled into a report, which provides instant feedback to the students on their daily activity levels. Access *ACTIVITYGRAM* from the Main Menu.

1. To start a New *ACTIVITYGRAM*, click the New icon.
2. To Look over, Change, or Add to an existing *ACTIVITYGRAM*, select the *ACTIVITYGRAM* (by name and/or date) from the on-screen list, then click the Open icon.

3. To Remove an *ACTIVITYGRAM* from the on-screen list, click on the appropriate *ACTIVITYGRAM*, then press the Delete icon.

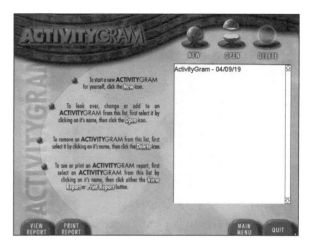

ACTIVITYGRAM menu screen.

Entering Information

The *ACTIVITYGRAM* screen consists of a grid divided into half-hour segments—from 7 AM to 11 PM. To enter information, instruct your students to follow these steps.

- In order for *ACTIVITYGRAM* to provide feedback to students on their activity levels, students need to enter information for a two or three day period. One of those days must be a non-school day. Select either School Day 1, School Day 2, or Non-School Day button.
- Select the appropriate time by clicking on the half-hour time segment. (Note that the clock on the right side of the screen reflects the chosen time).
- From the pyramid at the top of the screen, students select an activity category. A list of appropriate activities is displayed onscreen.
- Then, select an activity from this submenu.
- Click on an intensity level (rest, light, medium, or hard) for that activity.
- Have the student indicate whether he or she participated in that activity Some or All of the time for that half-hour segment.
- Finally, the student selects the I'm Done button. The activity is now recorded in the grid.
- Students must provide an entry for each half-hour segment in the grid.

For multiple entries of the same activity (if the student performed that activity for more than a half-

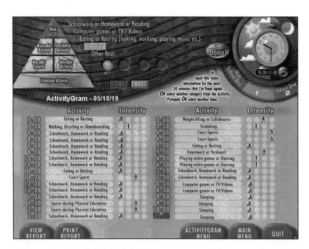

Opened *ACTIVITYGRAM* screen.

hour), have the student double click the I'm Done button.

To correct an entry, click on the time segment, and reenter the information.

View or Print an *ACTIVITYGRAM* Report

Students view results of their activity level via the *ACTIVITYGRAM* report. Also printed are recommendations for improving their levels of activity. See page 54 for an example of the report.

Technical Support

If you are in need of software technical support for your *FITNESSGRAM* software, please contact Human Kinetics. When you call, fax, or e-mail, please provide the following information:

- the type of hardware you are using,
- the version of the software you are currently using,
- the exact wording of the error message(s) or the message number(s) appearing onscreen,
- a complete description of what happened and what you were doing when the error message appeared, and
- an explanation of how you tried to solve the problem.

Human Kinetics Technical Support

- Phone: 217-351-5076 Monday through Friday (excluding holidays) between 8:00 AM and 5:00 PM (CST).
- Fax: 217-351-2674
- E-mail: **support@hkusa.com**

License Agreement

NOTICE TO USER

The installation and use of this product indicates you understand and accept the following terms and conditions. This license shall supersede any verbal or prior verbal or written, statement or agreement to the contrary. This Human Kinetics End User License Agreement accompanies a Human Kinetics software product and related explanatory written materials ("Software"). The term "Software" shall also include any upgrades, modified versions or updates of the Software licensed to you by Human Kinetics.

If you do not understand or accept these terms, or your local regulations prohibit "after sale" license agreements or limited disclaimers, you must cease and desist using this product immediately. Copyright laws supersede all local regulations.

Operating License

You are permitted to use the software only at a single address or building (the site). At the site the software may be used on one or more computers separately or as part of a local area network as long as the network is only within the site. Any violation immediately cancels all distribution rights.

Copyright

Software is owned by The Cooper Institute for Aerobics Research and is published and distributed by Human Kinetics. The software structure, organization and code are valuable trade secrets. The Software is also protected by United States Copyright Law and International Treaty provisions. You agree not to modify, adapt, translate, reverse engineer, decompile, disassemble, or otherwise attempt to discover the source code of the Software. You may use trademarks only to identify printed output produced by the Software, in accordance with accepted trademark practice, including identification of trademark owner's name. Such use of any trademark does not give you any rights of ownership in that trademark. Except as stated above, this Agreement does not grant you any intellectual property rights in the Software.

Liability Disclaimer

This product and/or license is provided exclusively by Human Kinetics on an "as is" basis, without any representation or warranty of any kind, either express or implied, including without limitation any representations or endorsements regarding the use of, the results of, or performance of the product, its appropriateness, accuracy, reliability, or correctness. The entire risk as to the use of this product is assumed by the user and/or licensee. Human Kinetics does not assume liability for the use of this product beyond the original purchase price. In no event will Human Kinetics or The Cooper Institute for Aerobics Research be liable for additional direct or indirect damages including any lost profits, lost savings, or other incidental or consequential damages arising from any defects, or the use or inability to use this product, even if Human Kinetics or The Cooper Institute for Aerobics Research has been advised of the possibility of such damages.

Restrictions

You may not use, copy, modify, translate, or transfer the product or any copy except as expressly defined in this agreement. You may not attempt to unlock or bypass any copy protection or authentication algorithm utilized by this product. You may not remove or modify any copyright notice, nor any "about" dialog or the method by which it may be invoked.

Backup and Transfer

You may make one copy of the software for archive purposes. You may not transfer this software to other schools, districts, institutions, clinics, hospitals, fitness facilities, or individuals.

Terms

This license is effective until terminated. You may terminate it by destroying the complete product and all copies thereof. This license will also terminate if you fail to comply with any terms or conditions of this agreement. You agree upon such termination to destroy all copies of the software and of the documentation, or return them to Human Kinetics for disposal.

Other Rights and Restrictions

All other rights and restrictions not specifically granted in this license are reserved by Human Kinetics.

More About
FITNESSGRAM
and the
American Fitness Alliance

FITNESSGRAM provides the physical fitness-testing component that's necessary for a successful health-related fitness education program. Once you know students' level of physical fitness and have identified their fitness goals, you can implement a fitness education program that will help them achieve those goals and learn healthy habits that will benefit them throughout their lives.

The American Fitness Alliance (AFA) Youth Fitness Resource Center is a collaborative effort of the American Alliance for Health, Physical Education, Recreation and Dance (AAHPERD), The Cooper Institute for Aerobics Research (CIAR), and Human Kinetics. AFA's objective is to improve young people's fitness and health by promoting physical activity and other healthy behaviors. We will achieve this objective by being a national resource center for fitness and activity-related products and services and by creating new programs to promote physical activity and fitness throughout life.

In addition to *FITNESSGRAM*, American Fitness Alliance resources include the following:

- *Physical Best*, the educational component of a comprehensive health-related physical fitness education program, is designed to support existing curriculums and enable teachers to help students meet NASPE's health-related fitness standards. In addition to a teacher's guide and activity guides for elementary and secondary levels, *Physical Best* includes educational workshops (available through AAHPERD) that enable teachers to become certified as Physical Best Health-Fitness Specialists.

- *The Brockport Physical Fitness Test* is a national test developed specifically for youths with disabilities. Like *FITNESSGRAM*, it's a complete set of resources for implementing this testing program.

- *FitSmart*, the first national test designed to assess high school students' knowledge of concepts and principles of physical fitness, includes a test manual and related software.

- Additional AFA resources are being produced to help you develop quality health-related physical activity programs.

Look for the latest information about AFA products and services on our website at **www.americanfitness.net.** And you can call toll-free to talk to us directly at 800-747-4457, extension *2407* or *2408*.

American Fitness Alliance

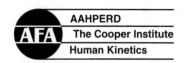

Youth Fitness Resource Center